Dementia Care Mapping
Experience and insights into practice

Edited by
Dawn Brooker, Paul Edwards and Sue Benson

Dementia Care Mapping
Experience and insights into practice

First published in 2004 by
Hawker Publications Ltd
2nd Floor, Culvert House
Culvert Road
London SW11 5DH
Tel 020 7720 2108, Fax 020 7498 3023
www.hawkerpublications.com
info@hawkerpublications.com

British Library Cataloguing in Public Data
A catalogue record for this book is available from the British Library

ISBN 1 874790 75 2

Designed by Andrew Chapman • design@thoughtplay.com

Printed and bound in Great Britain by Premier Press, Southend-on-Sea

Cover photograph by Sue Benson, taken at the Bradbury Centre, Shepperton (AgeCare)

i Contents

ii Foreword

JOHN WATTIS

Dementia Care Mapping (DCM) owes a lot to Tom Kitwood's concerns about the minute particulars of how we all interact with people with dementia. It provides a tool for improving relationships with people whose capacity to relate is impaired by many disabilities, including disabilities in memory, communication and sometimes self care. It recognises the central importance of interpersonal relationships in dementia care and provides an excellent framework for examining those relationships and how they can be improved. DCM started from a profound vision of the importance of the individual personhood of people with dementia. Tom argued that the understanding of dementia as just a consequence of neuropathological change was deeply flawed. Such a reductionist approach failed to acknowledge the layers of suffering and handicap that were added to neurologically determined disabilities by the way other people reacted to the person with dementia. In DCM we were given a robust way of seeing what such common and inappropriate reactions were doing to damage people with dementia. I am fortunate to have opportunities to meet people with dementia and those who live with them or work with them on a regular basis. I never fail to be touched when a member of staff responds appropriately 'person to person' to someone living with dementia. The quality of such interactions is beautiful and memorable. DCM is a way of making such interactions explicit.

It also makes explicit poor quality interactions and relationships and provides a tool for changing them. I still cringe when I see old people with dementia neglected or invalidated by inappropriate care or remarks. This happens much less than it used to with people who specialise in care of people with dementia. Sadly it seems to happen nearly as much as ever in general hospitals, and residential and nursing homes. Nurses, doctors and others who have to deal with people whose dementia is complicated by acute physical illness rarely have the training or the time to take a 'person to person' approach. In the NHS **1** this is made worse by a culture of 'management by objectives' which often results in a task-centred rather than a person-centred approach. In the UK, the National Service Framework for Older People (Department of Health 2001) has "respecting the individual" as one of its four themes and "person-centred care" as its second standard. However, the means to achieving person-centred care are seen as integration of assessment, commissioning and provision of services. It is person-centred – but not as we know it!

Some management theorists hold that management by objectives (essentially driven by accounting systems and financial considerations) does not achieve the best results, even for car manufacturers. Toyota is cited as a company where 'management by means' produces unrivalled results (Thomas Johnson & Broms 2000). This is achieved by paying attention to the minute particulars of how work is conducted. It is also achieved by ensuring that all workstations on the production line relate to each other as 'customers' and eventually to the final customer, the purchaser of the new car. Production line workers are seen as individuals who can and do contribute to continuous quality improvement, not as cogs in the machine. It is remarkable that similar ideas emerge from dementia care and management theory.

DCM and its lessons, if widely applied, would revolutionise the care of people with dementia. They would probably also help revolutionise society. Gandhi, the great leader of the Indian independence movement "reached people through direct contact, action, example and loyalty to a few simple, universally flouted principles: non-violence, truth and the exaltation of means above ends" (Fischer 1997). DCM, in its own humble way is part of the same struggle to ensure all people are equally valued. Enjoy your read!

Reference

Department of Health (2001) *National Service Framework for Older People*. Department of Health, London.

Fischer L (1997) *The Life of Mahatma Gandhi*. Harper Collins Publishers, London.

Thomas Johnson H, Broms A (2000) *Profit Beyond Measure*. Nicholas Brearley Publishing, London.

1 National Health Service – the UK's health service which is free at the point of delivery and paid for through taxation.

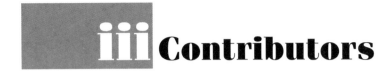 Contributors

CAROLINE BAKER is a nurse by profession. She currently works as a clinical specialist in dementia care for Walsall Primary Care Trust, UK and has been seconded to work part-time for Bradford Dementia Group as a DCM consultant trainer. Caroline works across all care sectors (health, social services, independent sector, voluntary sector, acute health) within the borough of Walsall to improve the well-being of people with dementia and carers.

ELIZABETH BARNETT's background is in health service management and research. She worked first with Tom Kitwood and then independently as a trainer in DCM, and is currently research development associate in the School of Health and Social Welfare at the Open University in the UK.

DIANE BEAVIS is a specialist nurse for the Alzheimer's Medication Service and is employed by the North Dorset Primary Care Trust, UK. Diane also leads the Practice Development Unit for Elderly Mental Health, which involves co-ordinating service-wide developments, implementing training events and advising on individual projects.

VERA BIDDER is a nursing assistant at Blackberry Hill Hospital, Bristol, UK, currently working for a National Vocational Qualification Level 3 Award.

JACQUELINE BOLTON is a nurse manager for services for older people (mental health) within the private sector. Her previous post was senior lecturer in mental health at the University of Northumbria at Newcastle.

EVA BONDE NIELSEN is director of the Danish National Institute for Elderly Education (Daniee), Copenhagen, Denmark. She is a specialist in clinical psychology, elderly research and supervision, and Strategic Lead for DCM in Denmark. She has been initiator of and responsible for a series of national and international projects in the research field of elderly people, including many research projects examining the care quality for persons with dementia.

KATHLEEN BREDIN worked with the late Professor Tom Kitwood on the development of Dementia Care Mapping at Bradford Dementia Group, University of Bradford, UK in the early 1990s. She now lives in the USA.

DAWN BROOKER is a consultant clinical psychologist and has worked with people with dementia since the early 1980s. She has been a DCM trainer since 1995 and investigated the usefulness of DCM as a clinical audit tool as part of her PhD research. She is currently employed at the University of Bradford (UK) within Bradford Dementia Group as strategic lead for DCM with responsibility for the teaching and learning agenda, research, and the development of international partnerships.

ANDREA CAPSTICK is a lecturer in dementia studies at the University of Bradford, and course coordinator for the BSc (Hons) Dementia Studies. She has worked in Bradford Dementia Group since 1994 and is a licensed DCM Trainer.

CAROLE DINSHAW is a nurse consultant (mental health in older people) working with clients, carers and staff for Worcestershire Mental Health Partnership NHS Trust. She works within inpatient and community units and provides a liaison psychiatry service to the local acute trust. She is a DCM evaluator.

PAUL EDWARDS is a nurse by profession, currently working as clinical lead, person-centred care, for Charnwood and NW Leicestershire Primary Care Trust. He has been a licensed DCM trainer since 2001, and is currently working part-time for Bradford Dementia Group as a DCM consultant trainer.

JUDITH FARMER is a community mental health nurse working in Norwich for Norfolk Mental Health Care Trust, UK. Her previous post was in a day hospital where the team used DCM to improve the quality of care. Her current interests include the use of volunteers and PAT dogs. She is a licensed DCM trainer.

JANE FOSSEY is a consultant clinical psychologist, working in Oxford Mental Healthcare NHS Trust and Oxford University Department of Old Age Psychiatry, UK. She is involved in training and practice development within the trust and with general hospital intermediate care teams. She is actively engaged in research into improving care using psychosocial approaches for people with dementia in nursing homes. She is a licensed DCM trainer.

PENNY GARNER is the originator of the SPECAL approach to dementia care, and chairman of the independent charity SPECAL which has as its overall aim the promotion of lifelong well-being for people with dementia, in Oxfordshire, UK.

ANNA-LOUISE GOSLING is currently in the final year of her doctoral training to be a clinical psychologist at the University of Surrey, UK. Before this course she worked as an assistant psychologist with older people in Harrow and Hillingdon, London.

MERVYN GRANGER is a nurse currently working as specialist practitioner in community mental health with a multi-disciplinary older adults community mental health team in Renfrewshire, UK. He previously worked as part of a community nursing dementia team and as a dementia liaison nurse with an older adults' day hospital in Dumbarton.

CRESSIDA HAMMATON, writer and grandmother, lives in Norfolk, UK and is one of the trustees of PABULUM, a local charity, reminiscence-based, which gives person-centred support to people with dementia and their carers. She is writing a book about her experiences, the highs and the lows, of her life with Peter.

GAYLE HECKENBERG is director of nursing at Calvary Retirement Community, New South Wales, Australia. Her previous post was director of care at Sandown Village and Guilford Young Grove Aged Care Facilities for Southern Cross Care Tasmania Inc, Australia.

LISA HELLER is a nurse currently working as DCM co-ordinator at Sheffield Care Trust, UK. Her job is to promote and support intitiatives that sustain person-centred care. She was formerly a nurse for Darnall Dementia Group. She is a licensed DCM trainer.

ANTHEA INNES is a senior lecturer in Dementia Studies at the University of Stirling, UK. She is course director for the MSc in Dementia Studies. Her current research explores dementia services in remote and rural Scotland and involving service users in research. She previously worked with Bradford Dementia Group and is a licensed DCM trainer.

IAN JAMES is a consultant clinical psychologist at the Centre for the Health of the Elderly, Newcastle General Hospital, and part-time tutor at the University of Newcastle-upon-Tyne, UK. Ian manages the Challenging Behaviour Service and has an interest in training and research.

MICHELLE JEFFERIES is a nurse working with older people on an acute medical ward for North Bristol NHS Trust, UK as a ward manager. She has been nursing for 17 years; her work has focused on the care of older people in acute settings.

LIN JOHNSON is an occupational therapist technical instructor with the Community Elderly Mental Health Team for North Dorset, UK. Lin was previously employed as a care officer for the elderly in social services, and before this worked for nine years as a nursing assistant in a dementia care unit. Lin is a qualified Dementia Care Mapper.

TOM KITWOOD was Alois Alzheimer Professor of Psychogerontology at the University of Bradford, UK, and leader of Bradford Dementia Group until his death in 1998.

DANIEL KUHN is the director of education at the Mather Institute on Aging, a division of Mather LifeWays, a nonprofit organization serving older adults based in Evanston, Illinois, USA. As a licensed clinical social worker, he has been active in the fields of health care and ageing since 1973. He is a DCM evaluator.

LESLEY LEE is a nurse and manager of a continuing care unit in Newcastle-upon-Tyne, UK. She is currently on secondment at the Institute of Ageing and Health, Newcastle General Hospital on a project investigating the impact of rationalisation of medication in people with dementia.

JACKIE LEWIS now works on a neurology ward at Frenchay Hospital, Bristol.

TRACEY LINTERN is a clinical psychologist working with older people in Oxleas NHS Trust, Kent, UK. She is involved in therapeutic work with people with dementia and in developing psychosocial approaches to care with staff. She previously worked as a research assistant for the Dementia Services Development Centre, University of Wales, Bangor.

LORNA MACKENZIE is a staff nurse on a day unit in Newcastle General Hospital, UK. She is currently working on a year's secondment in the Challenging Behaviour Service.

SIOBAIN MAGUIRE is in the second year of her doctoral training to be a clinical psychologist at the University of East Anglia, Norwich, UK. Before this course she worked as an assistant psychologist with older people in Harrow and Hillingdon.

LAURA MALLER is now in her second year of general nurse training.

HAZEL MAY is a state registered occupational therapist with a master's degree in philosophy and health care. She works independently as a dementia care therapist, consultant and trainer in Wiltshire, UK. She works in association with Bradford Dementia Group and Dementia Voice in Bristol in addition to developing dementia care services at the Royal Hospital Chelsea, the Milestones Trust in Bristol, and Dorset NHS Trust. She is a licensed DCM trainer.

GERARD MONTGOMERY is lead nurse for a community mental health team specifically for people with dementia and their carers for NHS Argyll & Clyde, UK. Before this he was a charge nurse in both hospital and community settings.

CHRISTIAN MULLER-HERGL is education adviser, In Via Akademie, Meinwerk-Institut, Paderborn, Germany, offering education and supervision to nurses working in dementia care. He is strategic lead, DCM Germany, and a licensed DCM trainer.

ANDREW NEEL is a nurse currently working as project manager in the Integrated Team, North West and Hucknall, Nottinghamshire Healthcare NHS Trust, UK.

TRACY PACKER is nurse consultant for dementia care at North Bristol NHS Trust, UK, and Visiting Research Fellow at the University of the West of England. She is currently involved in working with acute sector staff to develop skills and confidence in their care of people with dementia and their relatives. She is a licensed DCM trainer.

LYNNE PHAIR is consultant nurse for older people, Crawley Primary Care Trust, UK. Lynne has always worked with older people in NHS mental health services and the voluntary sector.

TESSA PERRIN is a freelance occupational therapist specialising in work with people with dementia and their carers. She has worked as a DCM trainer, and undertook her PhD research at Bradford Dementia Group during the 1990s.

MARGARET RANDALL is a diversional therapy adviser and gerontologist. In 1997 she was awarded a Churchill Fellowship to travel to UK, Netherlands, Sweden, USA and Canada to investigate provision of leisure activities for people with dementia. She is now involved in diversional therapy, staff education and DCM at Anglicare Chesalon Beecroft, and Calvary Retirement Community, Cessnock, New South Wales, Australia.

ROBINSON WARD, Mile End Hospital, London, UK includes the following staff who wrote chapter 9: Dr Jennifer Ford, specialist registrar; Ameena Corrigan, head occupational therapist; Melanie King, ward manager; Jackie Powell, deputy ward manager; Dr Joe Herzberg, consultant old age psychiatrist and associate medical director – all at East London and the City Mental Health NHS Trust, London.

MARIA SCURFIELD is a practice development nurse specialising in person-centred care at South of the Tyne and Wearside Mental Health Trust, UK. Since qualifying in 1984 she has worked almost exclusively with older people. She coordinates DCM within the Older Persons Directorate and facilitates staff development initiatives to advance person-centred care practices for patients, staff and carers.

SAILA SORMUNEN is a social policy researcher in the National Research and Development Centre for Welfare and Health (STAKES), in Helsinki, Finland. She is working on her PhD on DCM in Finland, and a research and development project using DCM.

CLAIRE SURR is DCM 8 Project Officer at Bradford Dementia Group, UK, working alongside Dawn Brooker overseeing the development of DCM Edition 8. Before this she was DCM Project Officer which involved delivering DCM Training and offering ongoing support to DCM trainers and mappers. Her first role with BDG was as a research student studying factors associated with well- and ill-being in people with dementia living in residential care.

PAIVI TOPO works as a research director in STAKES (Helsinki, Finland) and has a PhD in sociology. She has been working on ageing research for years and is coordinating a DCM development in Finland. She is also an active DCM user.

JANE VERITY is founder and director of Dementia Care Australia in Melbourne, Australia. She is an accredited professional speaker with an extensive background in occupational and family therapy and she is also a master practitioner in Neuro Linguistic Programming.

JOHN WATTIS is currently a consultant in psychiatry for older people in Huddersfield and a visiting professor at the University of Huddersfield. For many years he was a senior lecturer at Leeds and he is a former chairman of the Faculty for Psychiatry of Old Age at the Royal College of Psychiatrists.

JUNIPER WEST is a senior sister in dementia care (Specialist In-patient Services) for Norfolk Mental Health Care NHS Trust, Norwich, UK. She has an active interest in promoting the person-centred approach within her ward area, and using DCM as a positive team development tool.

BOB WOODS is professor of clinical psychology of older people at the University of Wales Bangor, UK and Co-director of the Dementia Services Development Centre Wales. He has been involved in teaching, research and clinical practice in dementia care for many years.

AILEEN WRIGHT is diversional therapy manager at Toosey Aged and Community Care, Tasmania; an urban and rural diversional therapy consultant; and an aromatherapy consultant. She was a winner of a national award for Professional Excellence in Residential Aged Care in Australia.

KATSUYA YAMAMOTO is technical officer in the Ministry of Labour, Health and Welfare in Japan and has used DCM in a geriatric health services facility and nursing home for about a year.

1 Introduction: celebration, validation and recognition

DAWN BROOKER, PAUL EDWARDS

Tom Kitwood developed DCM to assess the quality of the care environment from the viewpoint of the person with dementia. Tom studied and worked at the University of Bradford from 1974 until his untimely death in 1998, having established the Bradford Dementia Group in 1992. His contribution to dementia care practice has been enormous. His writing and his presentations inspired many. He brought together ideas from philosophy, theology, neurology, psychology, psychotherapy and sociology to develop a coherent model of dementia care. His contribution was recognised by his appointment to a personal chair in psychogerontology at the University of Bradford in 1998, and receiving Age Concern's Book of the Year Award in the same year for *Dementia Reconsidered: The person comes first*. In 2002, the Tom Kitwood Memorial Competition took place to commemorate his work in developing person-centred care for people with dementia. Paul Edwards' prose piece *The Dance* won joint first prize. As a DCM trainer Paul felt very strongly that Tom's work with DCM should be celebrated. This was the starting point for this book.

The issue of personhood was central to Kitwood's writing. He defined it as:

A standing or status that is bestowed on one human being by others in the context of relationship and social being. It implies recognition, respect and trust. Both the according of personhood and the failure to do so, have consequences that are empirically testable. (Kitwood 1997)

The development of DCM to empirically test whether personhood was being accorded or not to people with dementia, gave Kitwood's work a very practical application.

In the early 1990s DCM represented a breakthrough for those wishing to systematically move dementia care from primarily a custodial and task-focused model of care into one that respected people with dementia as human beings and was person-centred in its practice. In spite of Tom's death, interest in DCM has continued to grow. DCM training is now available in the USA, Germany, Denmark, Australia, Switzerland and Japan. The Bradford Dementia Group at the University of Bradford has continued to train practition-

> THIS BOOK BRINGS TOGETHER MORE THAN 10 YEARS OF THEORY AND PRACTICE IN DEMENTIA CARE MAPPING

ers, to conduct research and to support people using the method in practice. Under the leadership of Professor Murna Downs since 2000 and with the appointment of Dawn Brooker as Strategic Lead for DCM in 2001, DCM has continued to flourish.

There are around 35 DCM trainers and approximately four thousand people trained at basic level worldwide. The literature and research interest in DCM continues to grow. As part of the celebration of the tenth anniversary of Bradford Dementia Group, we particularly wanted to celebrate the lasting legacy of DCM that Tom's work made possible.

Tom's personal association with the *Journal of Dementia Care* (*JDC*) and the association between JDC and Bradford Dementia Group has been a long and fruitful one. A key member of the advisory board from the start, Tom wrote an article for the first issue of *JDC* in 1993 whose title – "Discover the person, not the disease" – helped to set the tone and purpose of the journal thereafter. Over the next ten years he and others contributed many articles about both theory and practice of DCM; these were published in *JDC* and are collected here to make up the larger part of this book.

The book's other major component is a series of snapshots of mapping data from the UK and other countries. Following the advanced DCM course in the UK in May 2002, mappers from across the world were encouraged to send a short piece of data and a brief description of how they were using the tool. The exercise was not designed to be a large investigation into person-centred care across different cultures. We simply wanted practitioners to discuss how they used the tool, describing both their successes and any difficulties encountered in its application.

Above all, this is a book of celebration. Mappers who have found the method of benefit have offered all of the mapping data willingly. Some are new to the method, some have many hours of mapping behind them but all appreciate what this tool can do for practice and also for them as practitioners.

The last ten years have seen many changes in the field of dementia care. There are more people with dementia on the planet now. Medical science has made huge advances in diagnosis and treatments for dementia and continues to do so. Policy makers are starting to take quality and consumerism seriously and want solutions to their financial, clinical and moral challenges.

The greater awareness that DCM brings facilitates more empathic care and a greater understanding in human terms of people with dementia. However, dementia care is still viewed by many as a minor parochial problem. Services for people with dementia still lack the funding to make person-centred care a reality for all. The truth is that in ten years we have only scratched the surface of these challenges. Excellent work has been achieved but often in isolated pockets rather than in whole systems. There has been little political commitment to developing dementia care and many projects around the world are seen as just that – projects. The gap between running a DCM project in an organisation and delivering person-centred care across a whole organisation can appear enormous at times.

There are many examples of how DCM has made a difference, a small taste of which is captured in this book. There is a need for a stronger voice for person-centred care and DCM. Person-centred care is maturing and becoming much more defined than before; the language of DCM is much more commonplace and acceptable. Concepts of well- and ill-being are established in care work now and form part of assessment and care in many organisations in the UK.

The impact of person-centred care is becoming more measurable and desirable for service planners and deliverers. There is a growing business case for developing person-centred care. Care providers know that developing staff skills, and working in a truly person-centred way that values all relationships, helps with staff retention and recruitment. Ultimately this can reduce costs in terms of sickness and stress. Independent care providers need to maintain financial stability – being able to demonstrate quality does much to raise the profile of an organisation. Clinical audits and governance are important with health and social care arenas. Various different health audit

bodies have positively viewed the use of DCM in the UK. This adds weight to this already powerful tool. It promotes its use and supports the underlying philosophy.

There were many who thought ten years ago that DCM would become just like a lot of other tools. Its main use would be for individual assessments and it would be pulled down off the shelf when it was needed for a particular person with dementia. The shelves and filing cabinets of dementia care practitioners are packed full of questionnaires, tests, observational tools and assessments. DCM has refused to be filed away. It has been a catalyst for driving change in practice and also has assisted numerous organisations to focus on their care in human terms. Mapping is a real and profound experience from briefing to feedback. We have seen it help change practice and attitudes on a small and large scale. We have seen practitioners grow with this new world of understanding and most importantly we have seen much less ill-being and more diverse and creative care opportunities created for people with dementia.

Although the tone of this book is celebration, this is not to say that DCM does not have its problems. Time and the resources to put person-centred care into practice have been major barriers to establishing DCM as part of routine care. Spending time focusing on the care of the least vocal and most disempowered client group within elderly care is an enormous challenge. As DCM trainers we are constantly humbled by feedback from mappers who have tried out the tool for the first time. We have seen new mappers moved to tears when seeing people in their care through a DCM frame of observation, particularly when witnessing high levels of well-being, the magic moments of care, or in DCM terms 'that +5 feeling'. This is the core strength of DCM, this is what makes it unique and maybe this is why people continue to use it.

Reference

Kitwood T (1997) *Dementia Reconsidered: the Person Comes First.* Open University Press, Buckingham.

2 What is Dementia Care Mapping?

DAWN BROOKER

I have been answering this question now for over ten years. I can provide some very lengthy answers, and some shorter ones. The type of answer usually depends on the level of knowledge that the person asking the question has about dementia care, practice development and observational methodologies. In this chapter I will describe DCM in enough detail so that you can understand the contributions in this book. I make the assumption that you know about person-centred care and practice development in the context of dementia services. Following an explanation of DCM I will outline the various chapters in this book and attempt to place them in the context of the other literature that exists on DCM.

I think the best short answer as to what DCM is all about comes from Tom Kitwood's final book *Dementia Reconsidered* (1997) when he described DCM as

"a serious attempt to take the standpoint of the person with dementia, using a combination of empathy and observational skill."

Dementia Care Mapping (DCM) (Kitwood & Bredin 1992; Bradford Dementia Group 1997) is a set of observational measures that can be used for a variety of purposes in formal dementia care settings. It was designed to be used in a series of developmental evaluations over time. Through a process of preparation and feedback, staff are empowered to consider care from the point of view of the person with dementia. On the basis of these observations, changes are made to care plans and practice generally. DCM can be used to monitor change and provides positive reinforcement for the provision of person-centred care over time.

Before DCM, measures of quality of life and quality of care in dementia reflected the very low expectations that were held for the lives of people with dementia. In reviewing the observational tools available looking at quality of care in dementia in 1995 I concluded that DCM was set apart from other tools by raising the level of expectation about what could be achieved:

AN OVERVIEW OF THE CHAPTERS IN THIS BOOK IN THE CONTEXT OF DCM THEORY AND DEMENTIA CARE IN GENERAL

"The simpler methods seem to suffer from the same institutional inertia as the hospital wards which they have been used to evaluate. They set their sights depressingly low. Inherent in DCM is the scope for identifying and recognising really excellent care. If the daily life of long-stay patients is to improve we have to evaluate against standards of excellence not standards of mediocrity." (Brooker 1995)

By and large I would still write that today. There is no other published method that identifies excellence in care from the point of view of the person with dementia. What I would write more about, if I was do to a similar review today, would be the importance of talking directly to people with dementia about how they feel and what they value. It has only been relatively recently that practitioners and researchers have actually started documenting what people with dementia say about their lives. DCM pre-dated this and has sometimes been criticised for not including the direct voice of people with dementia. It should be made clear that DCM does not work to exclude the voice of people with dementia but rather to reach those people who are too disabled, disempowered or institutionalised to be able to speak out. There are many examples of where the direct voice of people with dementia and DCM have been used as complementary parts of a pluralistic evaluation (Barnett 1996, 2000).

DCM in detail

Kitwood assumed a direct relationship between quality of life and quality of care in dementia and DCM contains measures of both. During a DCM evaluation the person observing (known as the mapper) tracks between five to ten people with dementia, known as participants, continuously over a representative time period (eg six hours during the waking day in a residential setting). The mapper attempts to blend in with the care environment as far as possible. Mappers are polite and courteous to all around and would remove themselves if they thought they were causing concern to the people with dementia in the care environment.

After each five minute period (a time frame), four coding frames are used to record what has happened to each participant being observed in that time frame.

• Behavioural Category Code **BCC**
• Well-being/Ill-being Value **WIB value**
• Personal Detraction **PD**
• Positive Event **PE**.

I will describe each of these in a little more detail (see also the charts explaining DCM coding, set out in Appendix 3, pp120-121).

The **Behavioural Category Code** (BCC) is a description of the main behaviour that has occurred in a five-minute time frame, ie what the person with dementia has been doing. There are a number of guidelines within the method that help the mapper determine the most appropriate BCC. There are 24 BCCs to choose from altogether (see chart p120). BCCs are divided into different Types depending on the potential for well-being that exists within them. A Type 1 BCC for example eating, singing, exercising, communicating has a greater potential for generating well-being than a Type 2 BCC such as withdrawn, distressed or self stimulatory behaviours. The BCC recording frame enables a picture to be built up of what those being mapped spend their time doing (or not doing) both on an individual basis and for the whole group. Patterns of different types of behaviour over the day and the diversity of different behaviours can provide a basis for improving the occupation and engagement of people with dementia.

As well as quantifying activities using the Behavioural Category Codes, the mapper also makes a qualitative judgement about the relative state of ill-being or well-being experienced by the person with dementia, called a **Well/Ill Being Value** (WIB), during the five minute time-frame. During DCM training, mappers are coached into observing signs of well-being and ill-being. Often these signs are subtle and non-verbal and sometimes they are obvious. Experienced dementia practitioners are often very good at spotting these signs and the training simply brings them out into conscious awareness. Prior to the 7th edition of DCM, WIB values were known as Care Values and this term is used in some of the chapters that were written using the 6th Edition. Well-being and ill-being are rated for most BCCs on a six-point scale, shown in the box above.

WIB values can be averaged to arrive at a WIB score for a particular time period for an individual or a group. This can be useful in finding out how individuals are doing in terms of their well-being relative to one another and whether change has occurred over time. Profiles of the respective WIB values can help identify whether individuals are spending their time in extremes of well-being or ill-being or whether they spend most of their time in +1. Combined with the data from BCCs it can also help pinpoint which behavioural categories are associated with the highest and lowest levels of well-being for which individuals.

BCCs and WIBs are recorded for each individual at the end of each five minute time-frame. Personal Detractions and Positive Events are only recorded whenever they occur.

The Well-/Ill-Being scale	
+5	Exceptional well-being – it is hard to envisage anything better; very high levels of engagement, self-expression, social interaction
+3	Considerable signs of well-being; for example in engagement, interaction or initiation of social contact
+1	Coping adequately with the present situation; some contact with others; no signs of ill-being observable
-1	Slight ill-being visible; for example boredom, restlessness or frustration
-3	Considerable ill-being; for example sadness, fear or sustained anger; moving deeper into apathy and withdrawal; continued neglect for over half an hour
-5	Extremes of apathy, withdrawal, rage, grief or despair; continued neglect for over one hour

(DCM manual, Bradford Dementia Group 1997)

Personal Detractions are any episodes of Malignant Social Psychology that are observed (Kitwood 1990, 1993, 1997). These personal detractions are any devaluing interpersonal interactions from care workers which could undermine the personhood of those with dementia. They are commonplace in many care environments. Care staff and professionals do not usually do these things with malicious intent. Rather episodes of malignant social psychology have become an unchallenged and interwoven part of care culture. Personal Detractions are recorded verbatim and are classified into one of seventeen categories and assigned a degree of severity ranging from mild, moderate, severe or very severe (see chart p121). Learning to identify and eradicate Personal Detractions (or Put Downs) is a very powerful part of the DCM tool – Chapters 11 and 12 describe them in greater detail.

Positive Events that occur in the care process are also recorded systematically. These include staff actions that appear to particularly enhance well-being. They might include examples where a person's needs are being clearly met for the first time by a care worker showing great skill. Another example would be where a particularly positive atmosphere is generated or where a deteriorating situation had been turned around. Positive events are particularly useful to feedback to show how good care can really make a difference.

Through the process of DCM much rich data is generated that can be analysed to monitor change over time both at an individual resident level and at an organisational level. DCM sits within an ethical framework of person-centred care which values all people within the care environment but particularly those who are most vulnerable. DCM should be used to empower staff teams to do a better job and not be seen as a punishment. This is difficult to achieve and much care and thought needs to go into preparation, mapping, feeding back and change management if DCM is to be of benefit.

Partly because of its complexity and partly because of

the risk of using DCM in a non person-centred way. DCM is only available through licensed trainers. The tool cannot be bought off the shelf. Much store is set by the quality of the initial training in DCM. DCM trainers undergo a rigorous preparation for their role. As a prerequisite for becoming trainers they have much expertise in the practice of person-centred care for people with dementia. The copyright of the DCM method and its training materials lies with the University of Bradford. As interest in DCM has grown, however, so has the need to provide standardised training in different countries. This has been accomplished by the development of International Strategic Partnerships with organisations around the world who meet the specific criteria for establishing DCM training and support within their respective countries.

The standard Basic DCM course is spread over three days with a written assessment paper which has a pass mark of 60 per cent. This course and assessment is essentially the same whether it is run in Bradford, Brisbane, Cologne, Copenhagen or Chicago. DCM Basic courses are organised by all the International Strategic Partners for DCM. These courses can either be open to all comers or they may be specifically commissioned by a care organisation who want to train a large number of their care staff at the same time. All Bradford Dementia Group Strategic Partners also offer DCM Advanced training which is particularly valuable for those who require a more in-depth knowledge either because they have managerial responsibility for DCM within their organisations or they want to use DCM in research. A list of strategic partners who provide training can be found at in Appendix 2 (p119) and is regularly updated on the Bradford Dementia Group website.

The structure of this book

Part I of this book charts some of the history of DCM. DCM was developed by the late Professor Tom Kitwood and his co-worker Kathleen Bredin. Their early aspirations for DCM and its development are described in detail in Chapter 3 and also in Kitwood (1992) and Kitwood & Bredin (1992). Interest in DCM grew quickly. The first training courses at Basic and Advanced level were offered by Bradford Dementia Group in 1992 and 1993 respectively. During the mid 1990s interest from outside the UK began to grow. The future German Strategic Lead for DCM – Christian Müller-Hergl – translated the DCM manual into German in 1998. Members of Bradford Dementia Group put on a DCM Basic training course on a visit to Sweden in 1998. Tracy Packer in Chapter 4 describes the visit that she and Tom made to the USA to deliver the first two DCM courses in the United States. Sadly, Tom died shortly after this trip. In spite of this, a strategic partnership between Heather Hill Hospital and Health Partnership in Ohio, USA, and Bradford Dementia Group was established and DCM training has been available in the States since this time. Tracy Packer's chapter also serves as an obituary to Tom's two DCM role-

play characters, Richard and David, who did much within the early DCM courses to bring the method to life.

With larger numbers of people trained and the method being imported into other countries, it was necessary to put a framework on training and competencies in an effort to maintain the quality and integrity of DCM. This is described in Chapter 5 by Anthea Innes, Andrea Capstick and Claire Surr. Chapter 6 provides an overview of DCM in its 'post-Kitwood' era and sets out thoughts for the future of DCM, in particular the Eighth Edition (DCM 8). It is expected that the revised edition (DCM 8) will be launched in the UK in 2005.

Examples of DCM in practice development in the UK are provided by Elizabeth Barnett, Jane Fossey, and the Robinson Ward team in Part II. There have been many successful accounts on implementing DCM. Further examples of using DCM to improve the quality of care practice have been published by Wilkinson (1993), Fox (1995), Moyes & Christie (1998a,b), Williams & Rees (1997), Brooker et al (1998), Barnett (2000), Martin & Younger (2001), Agger & Bonde Nielsen (2001), Wylie et al (2002) and Brooker (2003).

Most DCM practitioners know that sometimes DCM has the power to do more damage than good. There are many practitioners who have experienced some difficulties. The essential lesson that has been learned over the past ten years is that for DCM to be a success then it needs to be part of a whole systems approach to developing a culture of person-centred care. Organisations that have disempowered staff or have little in the way of developmental frameworks can struggle to implement DCM. Areas committed to development that have clear and supportive supervisory frameworks, are more likely to implement DCM in a way that is beneficial to both care workers and people with dementia. Jacqueline Bolton and her colleagues from Tyne and Wear in the UK discuss their experience of having to take a good look at their organisation before mapping could yield fruit in Chapter 10. A similar description of these issues is provided by Scurfield-Walton (2003) and Heller (2003).

Part III includes a number of chapters demonstrating how different aspects of DCM have been used to improve the quality of care for people with dementia. Diane Beavis and Linda Johnson in Chapter 11, Dan Kuhn and Jane Verity in Chapter 12 present examples and ideas for bringing Personal Detractors into conscious awareness and replacing them with more positive humanising care. In Chapters 13 and 14 Tracy Packer and Michelle Jefferies provide two case examples that will have resonance for many working in dementia care, where DCM data was used to build up a person-centred plan of care. In Chapter 15, Caroline Baker uses examples from her work with DCM to help challenge some common assumptions about levels of acceptable risk in the care environment. In Chapter 16 Elizabeth Barnett reflects on her experience using DCM to help care workers move towards a 'companionship' model of care for people with dementia in recognising the reciprocity of relationship that exists between human beings.

Many of the chapters in this book allude to the impact that DCM training and practice has on mappers personally. Examples of this are provided in Part IV. The first, in Chapter 17, takes the form of an interview by Tracy Packer with three nursing assistants – Vera Bidder, Jackie Lewis, Laura Maller. In Chapter 18 Andrew Neel, an experienced nurse, describes the shocks and surprises that DCM gave him, particularly when using DCM observations in hospital wards where he worked. In Chapter 19, Cressida Hammaton provides a moving account of her experience of DCM training from the perspective of a family carer.

Part V brings together a number of chapters under the heading of "Getting the most out of DCM". DCM is just a tool and like all tools it can be used badly or well. The outcome of a DCM evaluation will depend on the skills of those using it and whether it is an appropriate tool for the job. DCM requires a sound level of understanding and a confidence in practice. This is not something that is easily achieved in three days of a training course and much of the learning about DCM happens through practice. Feeding back the DCM results to the staff team is an aspect of the DCM process that many mappers find most challenging. Lorna MacKenzie, Ian James and Leslie Lee describe a workshop and guidelines for improving the quality of feedback in Chapter 20. Mappers across the world identify a need to have access to experienced users for advice and support. This need is a crucial one and over the last two years many regional forums and support groups have been established. The most structured example of this is discussed in the description of the DCM Regional Learning Initiative on Germany from Christian Müller-Hergl in Chapter 21.

One of the disadvantages of DCM is that it only focuses on a few people within the care environment. Chapter 22 describes a possible way of increasing this focus by including a measure of engagement as an addition to DCM. Maintaining the reliability of DCM is a major problem because it is such a complex method. If it is being used by just a couple of expert mappers then this does not present a real threat to the integrity of the data gathered. However, when many different mappers are engaged in mapping at different points in time, drifts in coding can have a significant impact on results. Claire Surr and Eva Bonde Nielsen highlight some of the problems and suggest ways that these can be overcome in regular mapping practice, in Chapter 23. Other papers on the psychometric properties of DCM are Fossey *et al* 2002; Beavis *et al* 2002; Woods and Lintern 2003. Another way of getting the most out of mapping is to ensure that the initial training is as positive an experience as possible. Paul Edwards describes the benefits of running a five-day basic course providing the opportunity to build in supervised practice in DCM as part of the course, in Chapter 24.

Part VI brings together a number of chapters that describe DCM being used in the evaluation of innovative care practice for people with dementia. DCM was used as part of a larger project looking at the effects of staff training on the attitudes and practice of care workers, described by Tracy Lintern, Bob Woods and Lynne Phair in Chapters 24 and 25. I describe the results of the ExtraCare Challenge Activity on a group of 20 nursing home residents with dementia where DCM was one of the main measures, in Chapter 26. Also, Siobain Maguire and Anna-Louise Gosling used DCM to evaluate the effects of social and sensory stimulation groups. Finally in this section, Tessa Perrin describes observation using DCM and her Positive Response Schedule of the effects of dance and movement work with nursing home residents with advanced dementia. Other examples of DCM being used in this way include Pritchard and Dewing, 2001; Brooker and Duce, 2000. DCM has also been used to formally evaluate the quality of life and care for people with dementia in long-term care (Kitwood *et al* 1995; Bredin *et al* 1995; Ballard *et al* 2001; Innes & Surr 2001; Kuhn *et al* 2002).

Part VII contains material not previously published elsewhere. It is a series of two-hour maps from Helsinki in Finland, Hobart in Tasmania, Nagoya in Japan, New South Wales in Australia, Copenhagen in Denmark, Dumbarton in Scotland, and Norfolk, Oxford, Walsall, Wiltshire, Gloucestershire and Worcester in England. This illustrates the diversity and similarity of mapping experience from different parts of the world.

This chapter and this whole book is a long answer to the question "What is DCM?". I have had DCM described to me variously as a Pandora's box, a can of worms and a treasure trove. Within the covers of this book there are the answers to many subsequent questions about DCM. One thing that usually happens is that new questions come to light in the process of the reflective space created by DCM. I hope that in reading this book you will gain further insights into your own practice both with DCM and person-centred care.

References

Agger C, Bonde Nielsen E (2001) *Kvalitetssikring af omsorg for svage aeldre: Pilotafprovning af DCM-metoden, Dementia Care Mapping, i Danmark.* Kobenhavns Kommune Sundhedsforvaltningen, Danie – Danmarks Institut for Aeldrepaedagogik. Copenhagen.

Ballard C, Fossey J, Chithramohan R, Howard R, Burns A, Thompson P, Tadros G, Fairbairn A (2001) Quality of care in private sector and NHS facilities for people with dementia: cross sectional survey. *British Medical Journal* 323: 426-427.

Barnett E (1996) *I need to be me! A thematic evaluation of a dementia care facility based on the client perspective.* Doctoral Thesis, University of Bath, United Kingdom.

Barnett E (2000) *Including the Person with Dementia in Designing and Delivering Care – 'I need to be me!'.* Jessica Kingsley Publishers. London and Philadelphia.

Beavis D, Simpson S, Graham I (2002) A literature review of dementia care mapping: methodological considerations and efficacy. *Journal of Psychiatric and Mental Health Nursing* 9 725-736.

Bradford Dementia Group (1997) *Evaluating dementia care: The DCM Method*, 7th Edition. University of Bradford. (available only as part of basic DCM course).

Bredin K, Kitwood T, Wattis J (1995) Decline in quality of life for patients with severe dementia following a ward merger. *International Journal of Geriatric Psychiatry* 10: 967-973.

Brooker D (1995) Looking at them, looking at me. *Journal of Mental Health* 4 145-146.

Brooker D (2003) Maintaining Quality in Dementia Care Practice. In T Adams & J Manthorpe (Eds) *Dementia Care* pp 240-255. Arnold, London.

Brooker D, Foster N, Banner A, Payne M, Jackson L. (1998) The efficacy of Dementia Care Mapping as an audit tool: report of a 3-year British NHS evaluation. *Aging & Mental Health* 2 (1): 60-70.

Brooker D, Duce L (2000) Well-being and activity in dementia: a comparison of group reminiscence therapy, structured goal-directed group activity and unstructured time. *Aging & Mental Health* 4 (4): 354-358.

Fossey J, Lee L, Ballard C (2002) Dementia Care Mapping as a research tool for measuring quality of life in care settings: psychometric properties. *International Journal of Geriatric Psychiatry* 17 1064-1070.

Fox L (1995) Mapping the advance of the new culture in dementia care pp70-74. In *New Culture of Dementia Care*. T Kitwood, S Benson (eds). Hawker Publications, London.

Heller L (2003) Using DCM in Health and Social Care Settings. In Innes A (Ed.) *Dementia Care Mapping: Applications Across Cultures*. Health Professions Press, Maryland.

Innes A, Surr C (2001) Measuring the well-being of people with dementia living in formal care settings: the use of Dementia Care Mapping. *Aging & Mental Health* 5 (3) 258-268.

Kitwood T (1990) The dialectics of dementia: with particular reference to Alzheimer's Disease. *Ageing and Society* 10 177-196.

Kitwood T (1992) Quality assurance in dementia care. *Geriatric Medicine* 22 34-38.

Kitwood T (1993) Person and process in dementia. *International Journal of Geriatric Psychiatry* 8 541-545.

Kitwood T (1997) *Dementia Reconsidered: the Person Comes First*. Open University Press, Buckingham.

Kitwood T, Bredin K (1992) A new approach to the evaluation of dementia care. *Journal of Advances in Health and Nursing Care* 1(5) 41-60.

Kuhn D, Kasayka R, Lechner C (2002) Behavioral Observations and Quality of Life among persons with dementia in 10 assisted living facilities. *American Journal of Alzheimer's Disease and Other Dementias*. 17 (5) 291-298.

Martin GW, Younger D (2001) Person-centred care for people with dementia: a quality audit approach. *Journal of Psychiatric and Mental Health Nursing* 8 (5) 443-448.

Moyes M, Christie H (1998a) Focus on each individual's experience and emotions. *Journal of Dementia Care* 6(4) 16-18.

Moyes M, Christie H (1998b) Structuring groups to make psychotherapy possible. *Journal of Dementia Care* 6(5) 15-17.

Perrin T (1997) The Positive Response Schedule for Severe Dementia. *Aging and Mental Health* 1(2) 184-191.

Pritchard EJ, Dewing J (2001) A multi-method evaluation of an independent dementia care service and its approach. *Aging & Mental Health* 5(1) 63-72.

Scurfield-Walton M (2003) DCM and Staff Development. In Innes A (Ed) *Dementia Care Mapping: Applications Across Cultures*. Health Professions Press, Maryland.

Wilkinson AM (1993) Dementia Care Mapping: A pilot study of its implementation in a psychogeriatric service. *International Journal of Geriatric Psychiatry* 8 1027-1029.

Williams J, Rees J (1997) The use of 'dementia care mapping' as a method of evaluating care received by patients with dementia: an initiative to improve quality of life. *Journal of Advanced Nursing* 25 316-323.

Woods B, Lintern T (2003) The reliability and validity of DCM. In Innes A (Ed) *Dementia Care Mapping: Applications Across Cultures*. Health Professions Press, Maryland.

Wylie K, Madjar I, Walton J (2002) Dementia Care Mapping: A person-centred approach to improving the quality of care in residential settings. *Geriaction* 20 (2) 5-9.

3 Charting the course of quality care

TOM KITWOOD, KATHLEEN BREDIN

Dementia Care Mapping (DCM) is a method for evaluating and improving the quality of care in formal settings. It is based on detailed observation, attempting at all times to take the standpoint of those who have dementia.

The story of DCM begins in the autumn of 1989, when Bradford Health Authority commissioned the evaluation of a 'club' for persons with dementia and their carers. In effect this was an extension of the Day Hospital facility to Saturdays, some of the help being provided by men and women carrying out Community Service Orders under the Probation Service. ∎

We wanted to make a 'pluralistic evaluation': that is, to consult with all the main interest groups involved with the club. Most of the information could be obtained through interviews. We very soon came to realise, however, that no method existed for finding out what the care environment was like for the clients themselves. The nature of their disability is such that they cannot make the kind of cumulative value judgement that is necessary in giving an opinion about the efficacy of a service. The common practice in evaluation of dementia services, it seemed, was simply to ignore the clients' point of view.

Not satisfied with this, we decided to develop a method that really would attempt to take seriously the experience of those who have dementia, however great their cognitive impairments might be. The method would be based on detailed observation, using empathy and intuitive sensitivity in a carefully disciplined way. The Leverhulme Trust provided the funding for this work to go forward.

Developing the method

There followed two years of intense work: exhausting, sometimes even heartbreaking, but also wonderfully rich and exciting. We spent many hours in a variety of dementia care settings: mainly observing, simply 'being there' - but also, where it seemed appropriate, giving a hand with the actual delivery of care.

Gradually we fashioned a technique for creating a highly

> THE AUTHORS CHART THE DEVELOPMENT OF DEMENTIA CARE MAPPING TWO YEARS AFTER ITS BIRTH

condensed record of the process of care (or 'uncare'). It involved two coding frames, running in parallel.

The first, Behaviour Category Coding, expresses in summary form what is mainly happening to each person being observed, in successive time frames of five minutes. The second, Personal Detraction Coding, is a way of keeping track of those tiny episodes in which a person with dementia is discounted or demeaned in some way; such episodes, although very significant, would otherwise tend to be lost from the record. The development of the mapping method was greatly helped by the fact that those who have dementia are far more 'congruent' than most people who have no cognitive impairments; both their words and their body language tend to show, with great candour and integrity, what they are feeling.

Each time we produced a form of the method we tested it out, and then adapted it further to take into account any new aspects of the care process that came to light, adding new categories or rules as required.

This development work brought many surprises. We learned that a place might have a reputation as a centre of excellence, and yet be very poor in the actual delivery of care. On the other hand, we discovered much about those places which have a 'special magic'; where the clients are generally full of life and well-being, making choices for themselves – and where staff morale is high.

We came to realise the weakness of 'commonsense' judgement, especially how this tends to miss the experience of those who are miserable but cause no trouble. We found that some methods of quality assurance are a mere facade, giving little real information about what is really going on.

Human reactions

In the light of such detailed and varied experience, we came to abandon the view that there are stages of dementia resulting directly from the advance of degenerative processes in the brain. Instead we came to view the dementing process as arising from some combination of

---

∎ For some minor criminal offences, perpetrators are required to work to give something back to the community, instead of receiving a custodial sentence or fine.

genuine disability and of human reactions to it. A helpful and empowering social psychology can offset disability to a remarkable degree; but a 'malignant social psychology' (and we have inherited so much of this from past traditions of care) can almost literally drive a person demented.

As our knowledge of the range of behaviour grew, together with the great variety of care environments, we were convinced that we had produced a method that gave powerful insight into the lived experience of those who have dementia. In its emphasis on process it was, moreover, strikingly different from conventional forms of assessment. We called it Dementia Care Mapping by way of analogy. A good map gives much information about the nature of the terrain, showing the routes, the outlines and the contours; but however accurate it may be, it cannot put every detail on record.

DCM in practice

Originally we designed the method to supply the missing part in pluralistic evaluations. However, very soon our emphasis shifted towards a more developmental purpose: that is, using the mapping data in order to give direct feedback to care staff and managers, so that a plan for the improvement of care might be generated as a joint venture.

DCM is now beginning to be built into programmes of on-going quality assurance, which accords very much with our overall intentions. The method has also found a use in research, especially since it gives a picture much more fine-grained than that derived, say, from studies of engagement. Experience has shown that DCM is highly reliable in the hands of skilled users. Furthermore, a strong case can be made for its validity: essentially its 'truth to life', and its efficacy in highlighting the good and bad features of a care environment.

We are very concerned that DCM should not be abused. For it is aligned to a set of values related to personhood, and a distinct view of what constitutes high quality care. Simply to see it as a technique, and to lose sight of the ethical position that underlies it, would be a dangerous trivialisation.

Because of the close and prolonged contact with the care process that it entails, DCM can touch some very sensitive nerves. A great deal of care and thought, then, needs to be given to setting up an evaluation, and even more to the giving of feedback in such a way that it can be accepted without hostility or defence. Above all, staff need to feel that they are supported and understood: that the mappers - whatever the findings may be - are on their side.

Although very good evaluations have been done by single observers, a team of two or three is certainly to be preferred. A team approach has been found to improve the evaluators' confidence in their mapping ability, and it tends to give the results greater validity in the eyes of staff. Teamwork also makes possible the vital process of debriefing at the end of each observation period. The experience of spending many hours in empathy with those who have dementia can be very draining; the mappers themselves need emotional support.

Teaching the DCM method

The first DCM training course took place in May 1992. It was soon followed by another, and another, and another ...

We were taken aback by the interest, and it seems to have grown steadily since that time. In part, no doubt, this has occurred because the method appeared at a time of heightened concern about issues of quality in all areas of service provision. Here was something that really worked, and it filled a gap that was widely recognised. Evidently it struck many chords with the experience of people already committed to the delivery of good care.

For DCM involves a view of dementia itself, and a view of the process of caring, that really makes sense to many people. Furthermore it is underpinned by a body of theory that takes proper account of the genuine findings of neuroscience, while not being taken in by unfounded myths.

We have now taught DCM to more than 400 people, who hold the certificate of 'Basic User'; of these about 50 have taken the advanced training, which leads to the much more weighty qualification of 'Evaluator'. The Manual has just appeared in its 6th edition. It is a very different document from our first production - thanks not least to the excellent advice and help given by some of those who have put the method to thorough test.

We sense now that DCM is settling down, with most of the earlier 'bugs' removed, and that further changes over the next few years will only be small. Bradford Dementia Research Group will continue to teach DCM, responding as flexibly as possible to all requests for help.

Looking ahead

Although these are difficult times in many respects, there is a new optimism abroad in the dementia field. The changes may be slow, but more and more people involved in care work feel that they are beginning to understand what they are doing; their skill is being informed by insight.

At the same time, it seems, there is a growing number of persons with dementia who, although they might score near to zero on any cognitive test, pass the final years of their life vigorous, alert and in vital contact with others. The use of DCM may have helped, in some small way, in promoting these changes. They are part of a new culture of dementia care.

• Published in *JDC*, May/June 1994.

4 The worldwide spread of the new culture of care

TRACY PACKER

Imagine the scene: you are strolling around a beautiful garden, arm in arm with a lady you are meeting for the first time. She welcomed you warmly and invited you into a garden with which she is very familiar. It is filled with azalea, rhododendron, honeysuckle and a whole variety of other trees, plants and herbs. She takes enormous pleasure leading you around the meandering pathways, occasionally pointing out a vibrant flower, encouraging you to smell the aroma of a herb, or stooping to collect maple leaves in an array of colours on this glorious autumn day.

As you walk around, you pass other people who may be chatting over a cup of tea on the veranda, or rocking gently on a two-seater swing chair. Occasionally you spot your friend and colleague also walking arm in arm with another lady who is showing him around the building.

This was the scene on a Sunday afternoon in October this year, when Tom Kitwood and I were welcomed and entertained by the residents during our first visit to the Corinne Dolan Alzheimer Center in Ohio.

The centre is a freestanding building on a rural, 150-acre site, which also houses the Heather Hill Hospital Health and Care Campus. It is a non-profit, non-sectarian organisation, which interweaves research-based environmental design, specially trained staff, and individualised resident-centred programming. Intrinsic to the care philosophy is the concept of homelife, a blend of relevant life history, current skills and abilities, previous "home" experiences, needs, desires and interests. All this is underpinned by the belief "that persons with Alzheimer's disease retain a capacity to feel satisfaction and enjoy life."

The occupational diversity made available to the 23 residents of the centre is intrinsic to the culture of the organisation, and definitely not a convenient 'bolt on' outcome to glamorise the hospital literature. Skilled art, dance & movement, and music therapists are integral to the team, sharing their skills and leading developments, without every aspect of these activities being seen as solely the domain of a particular therapist. Equally importantly, residents are not 'press-ganged' into an exhausting range of activities in which they are not interested, but have an individually tailored programme that is flexible on a day to day basis and constantly under review.

> THE LATE TOM KITWOOD WAS GALVANISED BY THE ENTHUSIASM HE MET WHEN INTRODUCING DCM TO THE UNITED STATES

day Dementia Care Mapping (DCM) course. This had made such an impact that they had invited Tom and I to facilitate the first Stateside DCM course, in which a large proportion of the centre's managerial, administrative and care staff were to participate.

Tom and I needed to get a sense of the overall care culture and meet the residents, in order to prepare last minute anecdotes and illustrations to keep our training sessions relevant to our audience. We needn't have worried. The course was phenomenally well received, with several light hearted moments. We were called upon to demonstrate 'frog-marching', explain what 'Snoezelen' meant, and enter into the true spirit of our role play exercises.

These role plays were to become the bedrock of most of the seminars, courses and presentations which we were scheduled to give during our three weeks away. They soon came in handy at the two-day conference presented by Heather Hill Hospital and the Cleveland Area Branch of the National Alzheimer's Association. What struck us immediately was the collaboration and equity of family carers with professionals, and the level of constructive dialogue between them.

Training through role-play

Our visit was extremely enjoyable, but Tom and I were not just making a social call. Eight members of staff from the centre had previously flown to England to undertake the three-

Cutting edge experience

Tom went on to inspire and enthuse his audience at the keynote address on both days, during which he delivered lengthy presentations on the development and practice of person-centred care. We were greatly encouraged and inspired ourselves, to hear papers discussing the use of music therapy, dance & movement, artistic expression and spiritual care. We were also thrilled that the Cleveland Branch of the Alzheimer Association was presenting a discussion panel that included family carers and persons in the early stages of dementia. There was an excellent consideration of the role of palliative care services. I was surprised and pleased to hear that a representative of the American National Hospice Association believed that people who are terminally ill and have dementia should not

Life-enhancing activities

The range of 'life-enhancing' activities available to people with dementia and often their visitors/family carers, at the Corinne Dolan Centre.

- Men's club
- Spiritual care
- Outside entertainment
- Music & dance
- Exercise classes
- Music therapy
- Gardening
- "Live Wire" discussion group
- Creative writing
- Flower arranging
- Woodwork
- Homemaking
- Sport & social games
- Intergenerational visits
- Photography club
- Groundskeeping
- Pet therapy
- Outings
- Art & crafts
- Literature appreciation

be excluded from hospices, but in fact should be, and in some places already are, accepted as much as six months before their anticipated death.

As with all inspiring training events, we wondered how family carers, people with dementia and professional carers could maintain their motivation following such a 'cutting edge' experience, particularly if they were returning to an environment which was very far removed from this ideal.

Deep commitment

During the weekend Tom and I travelled hundreds of miles south towards Lexington, Kentucky. One of our first visits took us deep into the Appalachian Mountains to the University of Kentucky Center for Rural Health. This is one of 50 federally designated offices developed to increase awareness of rural health issues. In an area of high unemployment, increased poverty and poor educational status, the center staff work within a framework of the interdependence of rural health and economic development. We were very impressed by the commitment and depth of feeling expressed by staff, despite being geographically isolated, working with a stigmatised population and undertaking vital work (see box, right) far removed from the high profile of the neuropathology research being undertaken elsewhere in the same university.

During the remainder of the week and between our own presentations we met a number of respected individuals at the University of Kentucky Sanders-Brown Center in Aging. The centre already has an international reputation in the neuropathology of dementia. However, we were particularly interested in a new PhD Program in gerontology. The Program Director was very motivated by qualitative research methodologies, and the changing relationship between elderly people and their environment. As three of the first year PhD students on this program were due to be joining us in North Carolina to attend the second stateside DCM course, we felt very optimistic about the future development of applied, PhD level research in the field. We were also very lucky to be invited to visit a new residential home where future project work allied to the University will take place. The Director of the residence has written a

wonderful dementia training programme for the staff. It is designed to maximise staff involvement and interest, and is loosely based on a "Golden Oldy" Hollywood film and therefore culturally very significant.

Tom and I were also able to spend a few hours at a day centre for people with dementia; run by lay volunteers using the 'best friends' approach. We had great fun joining in with their singing. However, we were both caught singing the British National Anthem with gusto, when it transpired that this familiar tune was an entirely different American hymn! This minor cultural gaffe (which highly entertained the other singers), reminded us that although much was familiar, we could take nothing for granted. (A momentary dementia-like experience?)

Our last long journey took us to the University of North Carolina in Charlotte, via Mount Mitchell National Park in glorious Fall colours. At Charlotte we delivered another DCM course, and one evening gave a public presentation that was advertised in the local press that day. Approximately 180 people turned up, mainly family carers, relatives and friends of people who have dementia: their thirst for information and knowledge was insatiable.

Finally, our role play characters (Richard and David = Tom, Olive = Tracy) journeyed a whole gamut of emotions

Kentucky Homeplace

This initiative attempts to address the needs of families or individuals of all ages, who suffer expensive and unnecessary problems because they do not, or cannot, access available health services. This may be due to lack of funds, health insurance, transportation, knowledge, cultural barriers or 'more pressing' life problems. Individuals are recruited from the target community as Family Health Care Advisors, and as they are from the community they serve in terms of education, dialect, values and culture, they are more likely to be welcomed than professionals from 'outside'. An important basis of these relationships is one of TRUST built up over a lengthy period of time.

Community Initiated Decision-Making (CIDM)

This strategy involves local residents who are actively involved across the state in an organised and structured process; to determine what they want from their local health care system, and how that system should be organised. Each CIDM Project is led by a locally hired 'Community Encourager', who facilitates the community effort to effect rational, informed decision-making.

Kentucky Telelinking Network

This is a 'classroom by interactive video' initiative for over 30 students at a time. These may be students of Laboratory Sciences, Nursing or Physiotherapy. The 'live' class is held at the main University of Kentucky campus in Lexington, with simultaneous transmissions, which can take place in rural classrooms across the state. This is a very practical step to encourage potential students living in Appalachia to consider undertaking a course of training, without the associated hazards of the two and a half hour journey back to Lexington through the often treacherous mountains (particularly in winter when many roads are impassable). This is also an excellent way to help allay the isolation which has been felt by students on secondment to the Center.

and experiences during the three weeks. Richard led a glorious rendition of Beethoven's Ninth, and shed tears after a particularly brutal personal detraction, Olive caused anarchy at a mealtime by feeding her careworker the crumbled remains of a melting chocolate chip cookie; and David raged once more to go home, almost breaking a door. On another memorable occasion David also flirted outrageously with one of our American hosts.

In acknowledging the subsequent death of Tom, it is also an important part of the process to say goodbye to both David and Richard, who (for those who met them) not only taught us something valuable about dementia care at conferences and on courses; but crucially, taught Tom much about himself. My willingness and ease to be involved with role-play now, is very much the result of Tom's persistence. Despite my early truculence and avoidance, I am beginning to understand the benefits of this process to my own practice.

This trip to America will always remain hugely significant to me. As a nurse, I felt that by inviting me to travel with him, Tom was saying something important about the valuable role of good nursing skills in dementia care, about clinical expertise balanced by sound methodical evaluation and reflection, but perhaps most importantly, about remembering to care. The trip was immensely valuable to both of us, with many people eager to share their experiences. Tom was galvanised by what he felt was a growing worldwide consensus moving person-centred dementia care forward. I learned much from our hours of conversation together. I shall miss him.

• Published in *JDC*, Jan/Feb 1999.

Acknowledgements

I would like to thank Bob Harr (President of Heather Hill Hospital) and all the wonderful staff at the Corinne Dolan Alzheimer Center and Special Care Unit; Professor Graham Rowles (Associate Director of the Sanders-Brown Centre on Aging at the University of Kentucky) and the staff and students of the PhD Program in Gerontology; Assistant Professor Lyle Snider and the staff of the Center for Rural Studies in Hazard, Kentucky; Virginia Bell and her 'crew'; the team at the "soon to be opened" Breckinridge Alzheimer's Residence in Kentucky; and last but by no means least Professor Dena Shenk, Director of the Gerontology Program at the University of North Carolina in Charlotte.

5 Mapping out the framework

ANTHEA INNES, ANDREA CAPSTICK, CLAIRE SURR

The Dementia Care Mapping (DCM) method was first piloted more than 10 years ago. It is now timely to reflect on the progress that has been made with this innovative technique for evaluating and improving the quality of dementia care. There is a great deal

HOW DCM HAS DEVELOPED OVER ITS FIRST DECADE, AND THE BRADFORD DEMENTIA GROUP'S NEW FRAMEWORK FOR DCM USERS AND TRAINERS

to celebrate; there are also a number of lessons to be learned. In this article we outline the history and development of DCM, what the method involves and the framework individuals can progress through.

How do you go about evaluating the quality of a dementia care service? This was the problem faced by Tom Kitwood and Kathleen Bredin in 1989 when they were asked to assess the success of a day care facility for people with dementia. The concept of 'client satisfaction with services' was less common 10 years ago in any health and social care context. In the field of dementia care it had barely been considered. Quality of care was determined largely by whether a care setting was clean and well-equipped, and its clients quiet, untroublesome and 'well-managed'.

The DCM Framework

Training courses in DCM began in 1992, making it necessary to have a manual detailing the coding methods and rules. This manual has since been through six revisions, incorporating suggestions from experienced mappers. Plans for an eighth edition of the manual are already under way. The DCM method continues to evolve, and since dementia care itself is evolving – together with our concept of what constitutes excellence in care practice – it will continue to do so.

Following the developments outlined above Bradford Dementia Group (BDG) has introduced a framework (see diagram). The framework has two aims:
• to encourage the sound use of the DCM method
• to monitor the progress of individual users, through maintaining a live register.

A basic induction/grounding in the method is provided through a three-day course instructing people in the person-centred philosophy of dementia care and the mechanics of the method. This entitles those who pass the course to map within their own care setting. Having achieved Basic User status an individual who wishes to enhance their skills in

the use of the method may produce a preliminary report providing evidence of mapping experience and competence in basic analysis of the data. The preliminary report is a prerequisite for the DCM advanced course.

The DCM advanced course provides participants with a greater understanding of the theory of the method as well as uses and possibilities of DCM for care practice.

The next step for anyone who has achieved Advanced User status, and who wishes to progress further and provide a full evaluation service to their own organization or on a commissioned basis to other care providers, is to undertake a full DCM evaluation and produce a comprehensive report to be assessed by members of BDG.

Following at least 60 hours' mapping experience a DCM

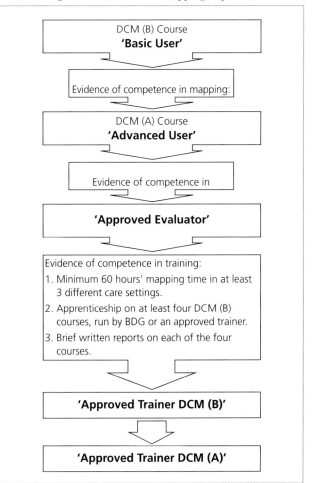

evaluator can begin an apprenticeship through BDG to become a trainer in the method at the basic course level. This involves apprenticing on a minimum of four courses and producing a reflective account of this for perusal by members of BDG.

The final stage in the framework is for very committed DCM Basic Trainers who choose to progress to DCM Advanced Trainer status.

The future

Since their early days both DCM and the person-centred approach have won the hearts and minds of many people. There have also been a few critics. To date, however, none have come up with any better method for evaluating dementia care. The greatest concern is, of course, that DCM is actually put into practice as a means of improving standards of care. To date there has been an imbalance between training in DCM and its actual implementation. There is sometimes a tendency for those who have learned the method to talk the talk, rather than walking the walk. Few care organizations as yet are fully committed to ongoing evaluation as a means of service development.

Inevitably, though, as external assessment and quality assurance monitoring become a part of every aspect of our lives, all care settings will need to be able to show evidence of this commitment.

DCM has now become an international method. There are approximately 1500 basic users of the DCM method in Britain, 300 in Germany, 20 in Sweden, 300 in the United States and a few users in Australia and Hong Kong.

A Primary Strategic Partnership has been established with the Heather Hill Care Institute in Cleveland, Ohio to enable the method to be disseminated to a wider audience. There have been many developments over the last decade, and many more are planned for the future. The cornerstone of the work of BDG and the DCM method, however, will always remain the same: putting the person with dementia first.

• Published in *JDC*, March/April 2000.

References
Kitwood & Bredin (1992) *The Dementia Care Mapping Method*, University of Bradford.

Bradford Dementia Group (1997) *Evaluating Dementia Care: The DCM Method*, 7th Edition. University of Bradford.

6 A look at DCM's past, present and future

DAWN BROOKER

Tom Kitwood provided Bradford Dementia Group with a tremendous legacy of work with Dementia Care Mapping (DCM). As time passes, the agenda surrounding it appears to grow longer rather than shorter, reflecting the incredible interest in the method and process of DCM. It speaks to people from all over the dementia care world and validates the work of many who have struggled to make sense of why care for people with dementia is so impoverished.

In April 2001 I joined Bradford Dementia Group as Strategic Lead for Dementia Care Mapping. Before this I had enjoyed a long association with the group and particularly with the late Professor Tom Kitwood.

On her appointment as the new head of Bradford Dementia Group in March 2000, Professor Murna Downs discovered that DCM had an enormous agenda attached to it, encompassing practice, training, international development and research. She appointed me to develop a five-year strategy for DCM.

A kick-start to my post was provided in January 2001, when 33 key DCM stakeholders including Bradford Dementia Group, DCM trainers, practitioners and researchers came together for a two-day meeting to share experience, insights and data about DCM.

The edited transcript and summary of this DCM Think-Tank (Brooker & Rogers 2001) is available from Bradford Dementia Group. I am indebted to the people who took the time to share their ideas and experiences. These have guided me over this past 12 months and continue to guide me into the future.

In this article I would like to update people on some of the issues that arose out of the think-tank and my work over the past year. It is also based on the growing literature on DCM (see Appendix 1, Bibiography, pp113-114).

Guiding principles

The aims of Bradford Dementia Group with respect to DCM are fourfold.

First, DCM should be used within an ethical framework of person-centred care that promotes the well-being of people with dementia, their families and those who care for them.

> TO WHAT EXTENT HAS DCM PROVEN ITS SUCCESS? HOW DOES IT NEED TO BE DEVELOPED TO CONTINUE ITS ROLE IN PERSON-CENTRED CARE?

Secondly, DCM is a complex method and process which requires skill and care in its teaching, its implementation within organisations and its use in research if this ethical framework is to be maintained.

Training should adhere to international quality standards to ensure the quality and integrity of DCM.

Thirdly, DCM has always been a tool under progress. The seventh edition was launched in 1997 after a long collaboration between Bradford Dementia Group and many dementia practitioners from many different disciplines. This progress continues and it is expected that an updated version will be launched 2003-4.

Fourthly, DCM training and the practice of DCM evaluations should reach as many practitioners and organisations who will find it useful.

What can be achieved with DCM?

The most usual way in which DCM has been used is the purpose for which it was intended. This is to improve the standards of person centred care – by means of a repeated cycle of developmental evaluations. It has been used extensively for this purpose in a wide variety of formal care settings, in the UK over the past ten years and in Germany and the United States for the past four. The collective experience, some of which has been published (much of which has not been), tells us that when the setting conditions are good the following is achievable:

• DCM reduces levels of ill-being and increases levels of well-being. In DCM terms -1s decrease and +3s increase.

• DCM provides both quantitative and qualitative data to demonstrate this, providing positive feedback on person-centred care which empowers staff

• DCM reduces or eradicates staff-generated examples of malignant social psychology (personal detractors)

• Over progressive cycles of developmental evaluation there is a shift in the focus of care to the most dependent people with dementia within a care setting

• DCM provides a shared language and focus across professional disciplines, care staff and management teams

• It has good face validity with (ie it make sense to) front-line staff as well as those responsible for managing and commissioning care

• Staff trained in DCM report that the training in itself has a positive influence on their practice

• DCM can improve job satisfaction which in turn can decrease staff turnover.

Organisational setting conditions

Any tool is only as good as the skills of the person or organisation utilising it. DCM is a powerful tool that can be used badly or well. In order for DCM to have positive effects there needs to be a strong organisational framework in place to support it. At the think-tank a number of elements were seen as important

• A practice development framework should be in place within the organisation. Reflective practice, shared value base, supervision, training and staff development should be linked with the process of DCM

• There needs to be a clear understanding at all levels of the staffing hierarchy of the philosophy underpinning DCM and the process involved in implementing an evaluation. Preferably this understanding should extend beyond individual care unit boundaries

• DCM consists of a cycle of preparation, evaluation, feedback, reflection and action planning. Resources need to be allocated to the whole of this process, not just the evaluation

• A lead person or persons should be identified within the organisation who have sufficient authority to allocate resources, organise the implementation, trouble-shoot, and ensure feedback is acted upon

• It is surprisingly easy for trained mappers to be insensitive to the needs of staff who are present during a DCM evaluation. Sensitivity to staff needs and those persons in receipt of care should have a high priority within any evaluation that seeks to improve person-centred care.

• Staff are particularly vulnerable within DCM evaluations where there has been no prior training in person-centred care Observing care through mapping is an experience that can lead to some very powerful emotions that mappers may need to debrief from.

• Giving feedback following a DCM evaluation takes considerable skill and those undertaking this may require support and supervision at this time.

DCM teaching and learning

The current structure of basic and advanced courses has served DCM since its inception. There are problems with keeping the training to a manageable size without missing out key elements of the method and the process of implementation. This is further compounded by the fact that individuals and organisations come to DCM with very different levels of expertise and skill.

Over the last 12 months the training has been updated and revamped. More weight has been given to the person-centred philosophy and feedback issues on the basic course. On the advanced course more weight is now given

to working to achieve organisational change with DCM alongside a more in-depth look at issues around validity and ethics. Where trainers are working with individual care organisations they are encouraged to tailor the training to meet the needs of that organisation.

Another option that is being explored is whether we should diversify the types of courses and levels of expertise. As well as the general basic and advanced, it may be that a research DCM course specifically for those only wanting to use DCM in research be developed. Likewise we might look at a course which concentrates on observing and recording but which does not cover data analysis.

Web-based learning for the basic course is also being considered. This would have the advantage of standardising the training material and ensuring that people could work at their own pace and from their usual work base. It would be able to offer additional support to those candidates who have difficulties with any part of the course. It is not expected that this would replace face-to-face contact entirely but it could be a useful addition.

How else has DCM been used?

Apart from what it was originally designed to do, DCM has been used for a multiplicity of purposes in different service contexts.

• Some initial work has occurred to develop DCM as a means of improving person-centred care in learning disability services

• DCM has been used as a focus for staff training interventions. Trainers have used DCM as a means for planning tailor-made person-centred care training and as a baseline against which to measure the effectiveness of training interventions

• It has been used as part of assessment particularly where a person with dementia is communicating distress. DCM can shed light on what might look like an intractable situation and in this way can assist in care planning

• DCM has been used as an outcome measure of care practice generally

• It has been used to evaluate the effects of therapeutic intervention or changes in care practice

• DCM has been used as a means of assessing the general quality of a service by some inspection teams.

In the absence of other tools it is easy to see why DCM has been used for these purposes. In my summing up at the DCM Think-Tank, I likened DCM to a large serviceable black garment which seemed to do for many occasions but which did not exactly fit all of them. For the future we need to ensure that the method is fit for all the purposes for which it is being used. One possibly is to adapt the method into a range of related methods to ensure its fitness for these different purposes. Taking the wardrobe analogy further we may end up with a series of garments that work well both together and in their own right.

What's new in DCM research?

Research using DCM has mushroomed in the last couple of years. DCM was not intended as a research instrument but it is being used as an outcome measure as I outlined above. It is in this arena that DCM attracts most controversy.

There is the thorny issue of where DCM sits methodologically. It attracts and repels in equal numbers those from qualitative and those from quantitative research traditions. It has a philosophy of involving staff in the plannning and feedback of evaluations, but it gathers quantitative data in a systematic way. It is too number based and reductionist for many qualitative researchers and too value driven for many quantitative researchers. Others revel in the mix.

DCM does not sit comfortably in the quality of care/quality of life taxonomy of measures that has occurred. DCM measures elements of both. Within Kitwood's writing is the assumption that well-being for people with dementia occurs within relationship. It occurs in the interaction between people. To measure the actions of carers and those cared for as if they exist independently of each other is to miss the point. Interdependency is key to person-centred care practice.

DCM has been used as a straight research tool without any of the process elements (staff involvement in setting up and feedback) that usually accompany it. When DCM is being used in a cycle of developmental evaluations of the same unit over time, then the most significant data is at the individual resident level. This data is rich and meaningful and the numerical markers simply serve to keep track of changes over time. This is the real strength of DCM data.

The data processing at the group level is much weaker. When DCM is used to compare different groups, it means that the group numerical data is the aspect of the tool that takes on most significance. Using DCM to make comparisons between units and care regimens brings out the second thorny issue. The way in which the numerical data is treated within DCM data processing at the group level makes most statisticians blanch. Group WIB (well-being/ill-being) scores and the Dementia Care Index calculations are both problematic.

For all this, there may be elements of DCM that make a good outcome tool. The face validity of the coding frameworks is very strong for practitioners and researchers alike. This is not a research arena where we have gold-standard tools for measuring life-satisfaction or well-being. We have many more measurement tools now than we did in the early 1990s. Many of these have been developed in the United States but US researchers are still very interested in DCM. There are currently two large US studies in progress investigating the concurrent validity of DCM against a selection of other measures.

My concern is that we utilise the results of this research to make the next version (or versions) of DCM the most fit for their purpose that they can possibly be. In order that the revisions in DCM can benefit from the fruits of this research I am very keen to hear from anyone doing research on DCM or using it as a research tool. I have a directory of on-going research which is known to me which I would like to develop into a more formal research network over the next year.

What might Edition 8 look like?

The current seventh edition of the DCM method was launched in 1997 at an event led by Tom Kitwood at Bradford Dementia Group called 'DCM: The next five years'. I assume this meant that Tom thought it would be good until 2002 and certainly there are now a number of things about the method about which there is a good deal of consensus for change. There are currently numerous research projects under way that will help us base the next edition on some empirical data. Given the outcome of these projects and field-testing and development time, 2003/4 is a realistic launch date for Edition 8.

One of the main problems for DCM practitioners is the length of time spent mapping and its complexity. Research will inform us how simpler measures correlate with DCM and what added value there is in doing a full DCM evaluation. Another question that can be answered from an empirical point of view is the length of time that maps need to be spread over to be valid, and whether continuous observation is necessary in all contexts. The challenge will be to make the measures simpler without making them superficial or unfit for the purpose in hand.

There are certainly some coding anomalies that could be simplified within the current method and possibly some codes that require expansion.

Related to complexity is the issue of reliability. In research studies it appears straightforward to achieve good agreement between two observers, but this level is much more variable in ordinary evaluation maps. Given the complexity of the method, drift is likely to occur between different trainers and different projects. The challenge is to build mechanisms to increase reliability in routine maps. Currently the equality of training experiences and a standard detailed manual are the main ways of achieving this. It may be possible in the future to post up test reliability video scenarios on the web every few months that all mappers need to code correctly (or against a gold standard) in order to maintain their accreditation.

The data processing and scoring systems need to be simplified and make mathematical sense. WIB (well-being/ill-being) value profiles will probably replace WIB scores. Profiles of WIB values are more easily understood by staff. The validity of the WIB score is doubtful as the scale of WIB values is unlikely to be linear.

Standardised computerised data collection and analysis and report writing is long overdue. Many mappers have developed their own programs for data analysis. The possibility of including standard software in the basic course is currently being investigated and this will certainly be part of the eighth edition. It may be that we have it available beforehand for seventh edition users.

The direct voice of people with dementia who are able to say how they feel about the process of care should be heard as part of a DCM evaluation. We are now in an era where the voice of the person with dementia is seen as important and needs to be heard directly where possible. DCM was an early attempt at putting the perspective of the person with dementia into a pluralistic evaluative framework. There are many examples of where the direct voice of people with dementia and DCM have been used as complementary parts of a pluralistic evaluation. DCM is not an alternative to hearing the direct voice but rather it offers a complementary viewpoint. The relationship between these two viewpoints will no doubt receive greater emphasis within the next edition.

A Positive Person Work coding frame needs to be worked out, developing the descriptions in Dementia Reconsidered (Kitwood 1997). Many practitioners are experimenting with ways of incorporating a record of positive person work within the current DCM tool and the concepts are now taught in the basic DCM training.

The international DCM community

International interest in DCM has increased at a tremendous rate in the past four years. Training and expertise is now available from the Bradford Dementia Group's strategic partners in the USA, Australia, Germany and Denmark. Interest has been expressed in introducing DCM into Japan, Hong Kong, New Zealand, Sweden, Finland, Norway, Canada, Spain, Switzerland and Luxembourg. An edited book on DCM and its applications across cultures by Anthea Innes is available (Innes 2003).

There is now a clear structure for setting up DCM training and support in new countries. The first international DCM Implementation Group involving all the international strategic leads is due to meet for the first time this autumn at the Alzheimer's Disease International conference in Barcelona. This is a tremendously talented group of people. That DCM provides a vehicle for this group of people to work together in the promotion of person-centred care for people with dementia worldwide is a legacy of which Tom Kitwood would be very proud.

• Published in *JDC*, May/June 2002.

Reference

Brooker D, Rogers L (eds) (2001) *DCM Think Tank Transcripts* 2001. University of Bradford.

Innes A (2003) *Dementia Care Mapping: Applications across cultures*. Health Professions Press, Baltimore.

7 A window of insight into quality care

ELIZABETH BARNETT

When we work with people with dementia our greatest need is to understand their needs. We design services and deliver care which we hope will be helpful to them. But how can we be sure? The impairment of short-term memory and other cognitive functions seriously hampers a person's ability to communicate a coherent judgement of the care they receive. Without this feedback, how can we tailor our resources to meet their needs most effectively?

In the health service our greatest resource is our staff. In partnership with the Bradford Dementia Group and the Research Institute for the Care of the Elderly, Bath Mental Health Care NHS Trust decided to try out a new method of evaluating the care delivered to clients with dementia, which would in itself contribute to the development of that resource.

The method was Dementia Care Mapping, developed by the Bradford Dementia Group under Tom Kitwood. The project was funded by money from the Regional Clinical Audit Programme. The aims were to measure quality of care in terms of clients' experience, and to see if this could be increased by giving staff the opportunity to observe the lives of their clients using the DCM method.

Dementia Care Mapping

DCM is a tool for evaluating the experience of people with dementia in formal care settings, such as day hospitals, day care centres and inpatient wards. It bypasses many of the problems of communication by using observation and the assumption that people with dementia exhibit much the same indicators of well-being and ill-being in their behaviour and demeanour as people without dementia. It is founded on a philosophy of the crucial importance of preserving the 'personhood' of the individual through positive interactions with others. The method itself has already been described in detail in Chapter 2.

The Bath DCM project

In Bath we decided to use DCM not only as an audit tool but also as an instrument of consciousness raising and attitude change. The actual experience of mapping is a transforming one, as the mapper watches the life of an

> **BY SHARING BOTH MAPPING AND RESULTS WIDELY AND QUICKLY, THIS PROJECT ACHIEVED IMMEDIATE POSITIVE CHANGE AS WELL**

individual client unfold minute by minute, hour by hour, and the method stimulates in each mapper a fresh understanding of the environment from the client's point of view. So we chose to train as many people as possible on the pilot wards. We chose them from all disciplines with client contact: nurses, domestic staff, occupational therapists, a consultant, psychologists, clinical managers, a porter, senior managers and two brave family carers. Even the Trust's chief executive came mapping – and he found the experience so fascinating that he did it twice!

Another significant feature was the speed of feedback. We opted for immediacy rather than depth of analysis. Instead of wringing every ounce of information from the data, and then producing a full written report to be fed back at a special meeting, we chose to map a given shift and feed back information to staff during their handover session. Consequently, about half-an-hour before the end of the shift the mappers would withdraw (armed with their calculators!) to a quiet corner to conduct an efficient first-level analysis and discuss the best ways of sharing their observations with their colleagues.

The fact that for the most part staff were involved in mapping their own wards gave an interesting extra dynamic to the feedback process. Also significant was the fact that each ward contained not only a strong contingent of trained mappers, but also a majority of other staff who had been involved in small group 'DCM awareness' sessions, so that overall the understanding of the method and what it was trying to achieve was considerable. It was not a case of outsiders (or managers!) 'coming in to tell us what to do'. Colleagues trained together, mapped together and fed back to each other. and as mentioned above, this was done on a truly interdisciplinary basis.

Genuine team approach

By incorporating the domestic staff and porters we were explicitly recognising the importance of their contact with clients. The response to this was usually very heartening. On one ward the domestic service manager would sometimes clean the ward herself in order to provide cover for her staff to map; and when the quality manager (a very senior nurse) of the Wiltshire and Bath Health Commission came to map, she was dumbfounded and delighted by the help and support in mapping that she received from the porter and two unqualified staff, who were already experienced mappers.

The active participation of the Trust's chief consultant in the psychiatry of old age was much appreciated by all staff. He enjoyed being able to spend two shifts mapping the experience of his patients and gaining an insight into the detail of their lives. And the ward staff enjoyed this opportunity to demonstrate skills and discuss feedback.

Benefits for managers

As interest in the DCM project grew, various senior managers expressed a desire to map too. The Trust's director of corporate development (who sponsored the project) led the way, and thereafter the directors of operational management and of nursing, as well as the chief executive, followed suit.

The benefits for them were that the method gave them a structure through which to understand the minutiae of care delivery as they observed them - a rare window of insight into the lives of the most disabled clients for whom they were designing and running services. They also shared with 'the purchaser' (the Health Commission for Wiltshire and Bath) an appreciation of the fact that DCM provided immediate outcome measures of service effectiveness. For the first time a Provider Trust could demonstrate the level of quality achieved.

The benefits for the staff were also evident. To welcome senior managers on to their wards allowed them to discuss their clients' needs directly and demonstrate their own skills. Although it certainly provoked a little anxiety to begin with, staff found it a rewarding experience. The feedback sessions were real opportunities for both sides to enter into a meaningful dialogue about care delivery based on a shared language (DCM).

The involvement of senior management also conferred status on the dementia care service, and those working there. Staff were obviously proud to be able to share their work-world, and moved by the appreciation they received. One manager wrote to thank the staff of the ward he had mapped, saying how moved and 'humbled' he had been by the gentleness of care he had witnessed. And the proverbial pin could be heard to drop when the chief executive began his feedback by saying how disappointed he was - yes, try as he might he had been unable to record a single 'PD' (episode of malignant social psychology)!

It's the way that you do it

DCM is about emphasising the importance of positive personal interaction for people with dementia. Unfortunately on inpatient wards the demands of caring

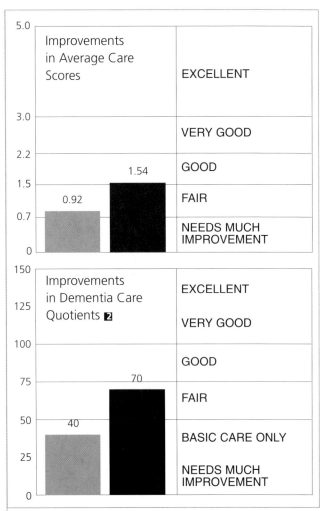

for people often with great physical frailties as well as neurological impairment, create very considerable strains on staff ingenuity in attempting to meet both sets of needs adequately. Inevitably the pressure is to complete those tasks of basic physical care (dressing, washing, feeding, toileting) which are crucial to a person's physical well-being. However, dementia care mapping highlights for anyone doing it the enormous psychological and emotional needs of clients which must be fulfilled if they are to preserve their well-being as a person.

In DCM terms this is represented by the difference between a '+1' experience and a '+3' experience of care. '+1' represents just a maintenance level of support of personal well-being. For example, if a person is sleeping, or if she is just sitting quietly looking around, then the scoring will be 'N+1' or 'B+1' respectively. In order for any five-minute time-frame for a mapped client to record a Care Value of '+3' ▪ it must contain some positive and affirming interaction with either another person or with the environment.

Hence any assistance with physical or personal care would be recorded as 'P+3' if it were carried out within the

---

▪ WIB Values and WIB Scores were previously known as Care Values and Care Scores; ▪ Dementia Care Quotient was an overall indicator similar to a Dementia Care Index.

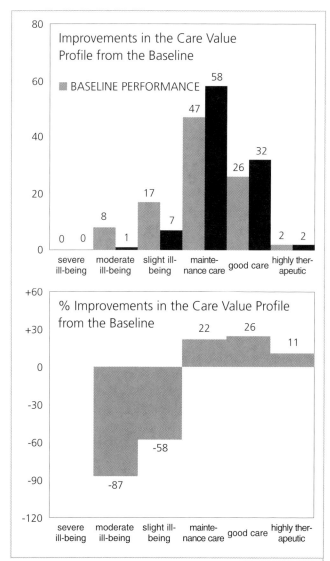

context of a warm and supportive interaction. But also if a client were sitting out on the patio showing evident pleasure in watching birds and flowers, then this would be recorded as 'B+3' (as opposed to 'B+1' for passive interaction with the usual environment).

When we came to evaluate the DCM Project we found that the best indicator of our progress was to be found in constructing a 'Care Value Profile' of each ward from the baseline measures taken before staff training, and then comparing this with an aggregate Care Value Profile of all the mapping sessions after training. We found that the '-3' (moderate ill-being) and '`-1' (slight ill-being) scores decreased markedly, the '+1' scores (maintenance care) increased, and the '+3' scores (good care) again increased markedly. Increases in '+5' scores (see below) were also present but more erratic. These changes were found to be highly significant. (See chart.)

That plus five feeling

In recording a Care Value of '+5' the mapper is witnessing a state of great well-being in the client. Often this is where an interaction is evidently highly supportive of a person's sense of self-worth, social confidence, agency (personal

control) or hope - the four global subjective states underpinning well-being in dementia.

A member of staff takes her coffee break sitting with a very elderly woman who cannot speak, but often utters repetitive little cries while looking round anxiously. Now they smile into each other's eyes, and the little cries become little laughs. Both persons seem to the observer to be enfolded in a warm and golden bubble of affection and happiness. After the caregiver has had to go back to work, the client continues to smile at the world, even reaching out a hand occasionally to touch those who pass by. She is normally rather withdrawn, and this represents a landmark in social confidence and hope.

When mapping we have all come to recognise 'that plus five feeling' when observing truly therapeutic interactions such as this. They are often found when the interaction is between the client and a close relative, or sometimes between clients.

In the first instance we are acknowledging the value to personhood of relationships built over many years, and during the project it has been very good to be able to share with visiting relatives the evidence of our raw data sheets: that the time they spend with their loved one is so valuable. We have tried never to miss an opportunity to share this information, and have always found it was very welcome. Relatives sometimes wonder whether their coming 'does any good'. We have been able to prove to them that it does.

In the second instance (interactions between clients) we are acknowledging that personal well-being is being 'passed on', so to speak, from one resident to another. For those of us without dementia it can be very demanding and threatening to open ourselves to the perception of the emotional needs of those with a dementing illness. How much more must it require of those already themselves engulfed in confusion? Yet where care is supportive of personhood we have seen moving evidence of this 'sharing' of wellbeing.

An elderly man was concerned for the choking cough of his neighbour, who does not speak, move, or feed himself. He reached out to hold his hand: 'Are you alright, mate?' And then for several minutes he persisted in gesticulating until he had succeeded in calling attention so that his 'mate's' condition could be eased.

Staff mapping this incident were deeply moved. And it was especially good to be able to point out that the first client was only able to offer 'highly therapeutic' care to his neighbour because his own well-being had obviously been so well supported. That is, in caring for him staff had indirectly been responsible for his being able to care for another.

Changing the culture

This contagious nature of care and well-being applies also, of course, to the relationship between staff members and the organisation. People cannot give what they themselves do not possess. For caregivers to be able to support therapeutically clients with dementia, they need themselves to be supported in their own personhood.

The DCM project has attracted great interest both from within the Trust and from outside. This spotlight on the dementia care service has been in itself rewarding. Staff have relished the opportunity to be involved in experimenting with a tool which is specifically designed for their service area, and which no other area possesses. They have also enjoyed the recognition that observation is an important part of their work, and the opportunity to discuss their perceptions.

It's good to feel valued

While it is true that giving feedback to colleagues can be daunting, it can also be a forum for the support of staff wellbeing. This is because each individual mapper is listened to and has the opportunity to express their point of view. For some mappers this is a rare experience. It is good to feel that one's observations are important, and valued by colleagues.

It was interesting that one of the wards in the pilot, after not being able to map for a few weeks over the New Year, felt aware as a team of a decline in their (high) standards, and set about re-establishing their mapping routine as quickly as they could. The culture of open-ness to feedback which has struck many people visiting the pilot wards had, in this instance, progressed to the point where 'withdrawal symptoms' were experienced! The staff perceived the lack as a decline in standards, but perhaps it arose partly from the absence of time spent listening to each other's perceptions.

Certainly from the evaluation interviews and survey it can be said that for the majority of staff involved in the project dementia care mapping has been a positive growth experience. Our challenge now is to take the method, and its philosophy, into the heart of our practice as an organisation. The newly-formed DCM Core Group which will be responsible for this, expressed its aim thus:

'To support a culture of person-centred care – both for persons with dementia and all those who care for them.'
• Published in *JDC*, July/Aug 1995.

8 A carer on the team

JANE FOSSEY

When Bath Mental Health Care Trust introduced Dementia Care Mapping as a service development tool in 1994, we were keen to involve carers in the process of service evaluation and be open about the practices on the wards. One carer, John Robinson, volunteered to take part in the 'Basic Users' course run by Bradford University for a multidisciplinary group of staff. John became part of the ward mapping team. Some four years later, I interviewed John about his experience.

> **INVOLVING CARERS IN SERVICE EVALUATION THROUGH DEMENTIA CARE MAPPING CAN PROVE REWARDING FOR THEM**

'I was pleasantly surprised that the ward staff adopted me as the ward carer and then I wondered what I had let myself in for. Halfway through the first morning I think that if anybody had spoken to me, I would have burst into tears, because I found it very draining and distressing but I decided to stick it out. It seemed very complicated to a layman, but I went back the next day with more of an idea of what it was all about.

'Looking back, I think the Bradford team did a very good job and it was made quite clear that if I found it too stressful I could pull out at any time or support would be offered. I managed to go through it and now I'm very glad I did.

'DCM was a great help to me, personally. I found I could relate much better to other patients when visiting my wife in hospital, and that stood me in good stead all the way through my wife's illness. I now feel happy to go in and talk to any of the patients and staff when I'm mapping or just visiting.

'I did find it strange to start with, giving feedback to staff about the things I had witnessed, because I wasn't quite sure how they would take comment from me as a layman. It could have been taken as criticism and at first I was very careful in what I said. When I found that other staff who were mapping were not pulling any punches, I was able to speak openly – both favourably and unfavourably.

'I think the staff accepted me because they thought it was good to have a carer who was interested and prepared to get that involved.

'I feel now that I'm giving something back for all the super care that was given to my wife, and I quite enjoy it. I found that at the end of a shift I'm mentally whacked but I still think it's very worthwhile. It's good to be part of the team.

'It's also helped me to meet a wider range of people. I've been asked to give talks to carers and staff groups, not just about DCM, and have enjoyed rising to the challenge.

'The most helpful thing for me about being involved in DCM is being able to understand dementia better. The most difficult thing is that sometimes I will see my wife in another patient, and that stops me in my tracks.

'This is where I consider myself very fortunate, because I'm able to talk about things and I do think it's good to have people to talk to who appreciate what I experienced. In carer groups, we are all in the same boat. You think you have all the problems in the world until you listen to some of the others.

'I'm not quite sure whether it would be a good thing to try to introduce DCM to a group of carers – it might work if there were a lot of carers in a similar position, but it's really 'try it and see' – it comes down to personalities to a certain extent.

'Before organisations invite carers to join in with mapping, I think it is important for them to know the carer very well. I don't think a lot of carers could do it – they would find it too emotionally draining. A method of presentation would have to be worked out using layman's language to introduce people to it before they do a course. The way I was introduced to it was very good.

'I would really recommend any carer to get involved. I can only see that it would be a benefit for them as well as the people they love. I would say if you have the chance, have a go, because you will be the one who gains from it, it will be an insight into dementia and you will be much closer to your loved one and other people than you were before.

'One of my favourite themes is that I was a carer at home for three years but I wasn't really 'caring', I was just keeping my head above water. I've learned more about caring since my wife was in full time care and I got involved in DCM.'

• Published in JDC, March/April 1999.

9 Clinical audit – a powerful tool to optimise care

THE ROBINSON WARD TEAM (MILE END HOSPITAL): JENNIFER FORD, AMEENA CORRIGAN, MELANIE KING, JACKIE POWELL, JOE HERZBERG

People with dementia in long-stay care settings are among the most vulnerable people in our society. Not only do they and their families have to contend with the devastating effects of a deteriorating illness, but they are also largely dependent on the motivation of care staff not only to provide physical care, but also to ensure engagement in activities and psychological interventions that are meaningful to the individual. The interventions should be targeted to the specific skills and cognitive abilities of each resident. Therefore care staff require high-order skills as well as sufficient time, if they are to provide a psychologically supportive and yet stimulating milieu. However, it is in long-stay settings that there has traditionally been a lack of staff training.

There have been attempts to overcome this using different models of care. For example, using the 'domus' philosophy (based on specialist residential care for people with dementia), an observational study (Lindesay *et al* 1991) demonstrated significantly increased levels of staff/resident interaction in the domus, compared with a long-stay ward. Staff working with this client-centred approach were significantly more satisfied with their jobs than staff working in the traditional setting.

Ballard *et al* (2001) carried out a study in of 218 residents in seven NHS continuing care facilities and ten private facilities using Dementia Care Mapping (Kitwood & Bredin 1997). The average amount of daily time residents spent engaged in activities other than watching the television was less than 12 minutes. While residents' physical needs are generally met in long-stay care, psychological aspects are often neglected due to lack of staffing, time and training.

The setting

Robinson Ward is a 20-bed NHS continuing care ward for people with dementia. It is situated at Mile End Hospital (East London and the City Mental Health NHS Trust) and serves the socio-economically deprived Tower Hamlets catchment area, in the East End of London. Nurse staffing consists of two RMN qualified staff and three nursing assistants on day shifts, and two qualified staff and one nursing

> **THIS CLINICAL AUDIT RESULTED IN TARGETS FOR ACTIVITY TIME BEING ACHIEVED WITH NO INCREASE IN STAFFING NEEDED**

assistant at night. There is a part-time occupational therapy assistant and sessional input from a psychologist on request. If, following assessment by the local dementia assessment unit, specialist high-level mental health nursing is required that cannot be provided by other local community services, a person will be admitted. Invariably, residents have challenging behaviour on admission to the unit.

In early 2001 the ward's consultant (JH) had received various separate representations from lead nurses, psychologist and occupational therapists expressing concern that there were insufficient resources to provide adequate therapeutic interventions for residents on the ward. In each instance, the person indicating concern expressed frustration with the lack of input from the other professional disciplines. It was clear that a blame culture was operating and yet all the professional groups were keen to promote enhanced therapeutic activity on the ward.

The service manager had arranged for the ward to undergo a Dementia Care Mapping assessment to support the service. The consultant convened a meeting of senior staff from medical, nursing, OT and psychology professions (the steering group) and it was agreed that it would be useful to audit formally the amount of therapeutic activity that was taking place.

The audit

We decided to carry out a baseline assessment of the amount of therapeutic activity each resident was engaged in per day, based on a week's observation and recording. There was little guidance in the literature about the amount of therapeutic activity that residents in a continuing care setting should optimally receive, but we all agreed the more, the better. We were surprised by the findings of Ballard *et al* (2001). We calculated that allowing for the amount of time nurses spend in undertaking physical care activities and nursing intervention for residents, the potential therapeutic value of which was acknowledged but not included, it should be possible to aim to provide an average of one hour per day of therapeutic activities for each resident (Standard 1 ■). A form was drawn up to

---

■ These standards refer to UK National Care Standards.

record therapeutic activities.

We agreed that only informal and formal therapeutic activities lasting five minutes or more should be recorded. We planned that three audits would each be carried out for a week, first before the Dementia Care Mapping exercise, then in the middle of the training (which was spread over two months), and finally after the training. Results would be reported in minutes per resident per day, corrected to the nearest minute. Informal activities were defined as interactions carried out by any member of staff to provide emotional support to residents. This category includes coffee groups, or general informal discussions. Time spent watching television was specifically excluded, although a discussion about a programme would be included.

Formal therapeutic activities included behavioural management counselling, multi-sensory therapy groups or individual work, one-to-one counselling, music therapy activities, the use of the reminiscence room, cooking, reality orientation and validation therapy. We also agreed that every resident should have a multiprofessional care plan, with identified therapeutic activities (Standard 2). The audit was discussed with the relatives/carers of the ward residents through the close involvement of the chair of the carers' group, who gave the audit his full support. The form was piloted to ensure that it was easy to fill out.

Results

A baseline audit (audit 1) was carried out on the week commencing 15 October 2001 and we found that the mean time per day that each resident was involved in psychologically oriented activities was 29 minutes (range 14-64 minutes). Audit 2 was carried out midway through the Dementia Care Mapping training on the week commencing 7 January 2002 and the average amount of time per resident per had risen to 49 minutes (range 14-90 minutes).

A third audit of activity was carried out after the completion of training and the mean time per resident had fallen to 17 minutes (range 1-30 minutes). The reasons for this were analysed and it was noted that the ward's OT assistant (who runs many of the formal activities) had been on unexpected sick leave during the audit period. The steering group unanimously agreed to continue to reaudit at regular intervals.

In a fourth audit carried out on the week of 17 June 2002, the amount of therapeutic time per resident per day had risen to 37 minutes (range 15-65 minutes), despite an identified failure of one key member of staff to record all activities that week. In a fifth audit carried out on the week of 11 November 2002, the amount of therapeutic activity had risen to 56 minutes (range 15-127 minutes) and in a sixth audit during the week of 17 February 2003, the amount of therapeutic activity had again increased to 110 minutes per resident per day (range 41-184 minutes).

The large increase in therapeutic time noted between the fifth and sixth audits is probably due to the purchase of some portable multi-sensory equipment, which enabled interventions to be more accessible to immobile residents with high dependency needs.

Standard 1 had nearly been achieved by the fifth audit and was exceeded in the sixth. Standard 2, which set out the requirement for a multiprofessional care plan to include therapeutic activities, was achieved in all six audits.

Discussion

Clinical audit occurs in real clinical settings and, unlike research, it is difficult to control for day-to-day variations in care and behaviour. Therefore our audit was affected by staff sickness on one occasion, and poor recording technique on another. Despite these variations, which are inevitable in a clinical setting, we have demonstrated a near fourfold increase in therapeutic activity for residents in this long-stay ward, over a period of 16 months. On reflection we feel that the Dementia Care Mapping exercise and training gave ward staff knowledge of a greater variety of potential therapeutic interventions. It is clear from the results that this intervention alone did not account for the continuing improvements that occurred over the fourth to sixth audits.

The steering group was pleased to note that the ward team had taken up the audit enthusiastically and was keen to carry it out, despite the extra work that it caused. They awaited the calculation of the results eagerly. Therefore we believe that it was the audit process itself, coupled with the team's commitment that brought about the desired results.

The original aim of the audit was to draw the attention of management to increased staffing requirements. The actual result was more optimal use of staff time, without the need for increased staffing levels.

• Published in JDC, Nov/Dec 2003.

References

Ballard C, Fossey J, Ramilgan C et al (2001) Quality of care in private sector and NHS facilities for people with dementia: cross sectional survey. British Medical Journal 323 426-427.

Kitwood T, Bredin K (1997) Evaluating dementia care: the DCM method. 7th ed. Bradford Dementia Group, Bradford.

Lindesay J, Briggs K, Lawes M et al (1991) The domus philosophy: a comparative evaluation of a new approach to residential care for the demented elderly. International Journal of Geriatric Psychiatry 6 727-736.

10 Stepping back to move forward with DCM

JACQUELINE BOLTON, IAN GEE, LESLEY JACKSON, DONNA MATHER, LESLEY POTTER, SUE ROBERTS, PAULA ROBSON, MARIA SCURFIELD, DORIS STEWART, CLARE VANDOR

Dementia Care Mapping has gained national and international recognition as a reliable evaluation tool to measure the experiences of care from the perspective of the person with dementia (Bradford Dementia Group 1997).

There have been numerous publications indicating the value of Dementia Care Mapping (DCM) as a quality assurance mechanism that enables improvements in the quality of care of people with dementia (Brooker et al 1998, Buckland 1995, Williams & Rees 1997).

While endorsing these values, we would like to share our experience that DCM alone will not bring about the changes that are needed in practice to develop a person-centred dementia care culture. This article will focus on organisational, professional and practice development issues that have evolved following the introduction of DCM as a quality assurance tool.

The introduction of DCM

In 1995 the Psychiatry of Old Age Directorate at Priority Healthcare Wearside NHS Trust introduced Dementia Care Mapping. A letter was circulated to all clinical areas in the directorate, offering a development opportunity for clinical nursing staff to attend the basic DCM course. Interested staff were invited to apply firstly stating reasons why they should be selected and secondly how they would propose to take the development forward. From a number of applications three staff were chosen, two staff nurses and an enrolled nurse, all having a direct impact on patient care. This was felt to be particularly important to enhance clinical credibility of the method and influence positive changes in care practices.

Following successful completion of the course the mappers – fired with enthusiasm – began giving presentations about the DCM method. The intention of these presentations was to raise awareness of Dementia Care Mapping and the potential impact on the quality of patient care, inform staff of the methodology and prepare staff for DCM evaluations taking place on clinical areas.

Initial responses from some nursing staff were fairly

> IT IS NECESSARY TO TAKE A STEP BACK AND ASSESS HOW THE PROCESS OF MAPPING AFFECTS EVERYONE INVOLVED

negative. They found it difficult to relate DCM to improvements in patient care and felt threatened by the evaluation method and the introduction of a relatively new concept. In addition, not all staff were familiar with the more recent developments of person-centred care practices. There was however a very positive response from individual nurses, other members of the multidisciplinary team, members of the quality department, line managers and purchasers, which assisted in driving the initiative forward.

Following an extensive range of presentations the first map took place on a 32-bed continuing care ward ◼1. Following the assessment, mappers organised a feedback presentation with the ward team. One of the aims of the feedback was to give the ward team ownership of the information in order to plan improvements in patient care. However, some staff found great difficulty in accepting the feedback, perceiving it as criticism of the quality of their caregiving. They dwelt on the negative aspects of the feedback, particularly the personal detractions that were highlighted. Out of the many areas of clinical practice which required improvement the ward team focused upon a small number of issues. This led to the mappers feeling frustrated and unable to bring about all the changes required by the team.

There were many incidents of personal detractions throughout the evaluation, including Ignoring, Objectification, Outpacing and Disempowerment. Most were rated as mild to moderate, but some Objectification was severe – for example, a patient in distress given a drink by a care worker who did not acknowledge the patient but carried on a conversation with another staff member. Some of the team were very defensive and unwilling to acknowledge the effect of personal detractions on patients' well-being. Throughout the feedback session the team also showed a reluctance to acknowledge any positive effects from the evaluation, and disagreed with the mappers about the benefits of this group activity.

The ward team also focused its anger on the individual mappers who felt alienated, isolated, and increasingly vulnerable. It raised an important issue of maintaining the

---

◼1 Long-stay ward provided by the UK National Health Service.

well being of both the mappers and the clinical staff. During this time the mappers sought informal support from colleagues, both mappers and non-mappers.

Later discussions with mappers from other NHS trusts revealed that ours was not a unique experience.

A new strategy is developed

As new mappers we had made an assumption that clinical staff would immediately embrace person-centred care practices, including DCM. On reflection, we realised that we were wrong to make that assumption and we needed to revisit our original objectives. We subsequently formulated a strategy which included issues regarding the management, delivery and development of new practices. DCM evaluations were postponed for a period of time to allow us to concentrate on our strategy.

As a result of this awareness an investment in person-centred care training for all grades of staff was made over a period of time. This was carried out in-house and included members of the Bradford Dementia Group and other experts in the field speaking to staff.

It was also agreed to train more mappers for support, and to widen the range of professional backgrounds to include clinical leaders, managers and educators.

On return from the training it became clear that there was a need to examine how the team was to move forward and to develop standards of practice in relation to DCM. It also became apparent that in order to develop as a group of mappers, offer support, discuss professional and operational issues, plan maps and develop personally, a regular group meeting would be required. A special interest group was established to explore operational issues relating to mapping, meeting for an hour and a half every month and looking at professional and development issues.

At its inaugural meeting the group agreed upon its terms of reference. Work began on an operational policy for DCM, which was distributed to ward managers for discussion with their teams. This also ensured a consistent approach for all mappers.

To enhance co-ordination and consistency, a presentation package for delivery to clinical areas was developed alongside a data collection pack for the mappers. As part of the presentation pack, questionnaires were developed to assess the attitudes and opinions of clinical staff regarding DCM.

A conflict of priorities

As DCM evaluations became an integral part of practice it became evident that there were a number of professional practice and personal issues related to mapping that needed to be explored and resolved. It was felt that more time was needed to address these issues and therefore meetings were increased to half a day each month.

One of the first issues to arise was the conflict between the role of an individual as a mapper versus the role as a nurse – this was with reference on when to intervene in care delivery when mapping. The issues raised were in relation to responsibility and accountability. While the team were there as mappers, they were also nurses bound by a professional code of conduct. Being a mapper, observing personal detractions and practice dilemmas relating to care delivery proved very difficult. Mappers felt very uncomfortable at times. We subsequently developed a clear procedure for dealing with unsafe practice.

There were also issues relating to the conflict between observing and participating in 'hands-on' patient care. Through reflection and critical discussion, the group were able to move on from this. The focus of the resolution was to consider the purpose of mapping. Mappers intervening in care had made the ward team very uncomfortable and had been viewed as a criticism of their care or lack of intervention.

Individuals in the group felt that in sharing these issues they were supported and could support others. The group offered a safe environment in which to explore issues and to share feelings about care practices and the role of mappers.

Other issues raised included those of confidentiality and informed consent. The group felt that there were areas of concern relating to the patient being unable to give consent to the map. Members of the group felt that consideration should be given to the code of conduct and in this instance sought to resolve the issue by referring to the chief nurse of the Trust, drawing upon his expertise. To assist in resolving this issue, it was agreed to introduce ourselves at the beginning of each map and explain our purpose. If an individual became distressed by being observed then that observation would cease. If the individual continued to be distressed by the mapping then it would be stopped.

Clinical supervision

Through this process there came a very clear indicator that clinical supervision was the way forward to facilitate reflection, resolution of the issues and to offer mutual support. The meeting was then divided into two distinct parts, one part for operational issues and the other for clinical supervision. There was also a need for ongoing training and development of mappers, which was addressed.

To ensure that these meetings reflected the professional and personal needs of the group a clinical supervision contract was developed. The contract covers issues of attendance, confidentiality, and roles and responsibilities of mappers. Within the contract is a clearly-defined procedure for dealing with unsafe practice and practice dilemmas.

Supervision addresses a wide variety of areas including professional issues and accountability issues related to role, personal issues, further training and development as well as the development of reflective diaries.

The work carried out within this group format has resulted in changes which have enhanced the experience for clinical staff and mappers alike. These have included developing the role of an observer, nominated by the clinical area being mapped. To assist this process, observer guidelines have been developed. The clinical observer has come to serve an important role in the mapping process as they produce very rich data and give excellent feedback to their team. Their feedback is included in the oral and written feedback that is given to the ward team. Some of the documentation has also been changed to focus the discussion and feedback to the clinical staff, reflecting the positive aspects of the map.

Other work has included a structured agenda for the group to assist the meeting in running smoothly, definition of roles and responsibilities of mappers in the areas of mapping, action planning and feedback.

An audit plan based on a three-year cycle, to evaluate the impact of DCM on patient care and staff attitudes, is currently in process.

Training and development for ward teams have focused on the development of action plans following DCM evaluations. Action planning guidelines have been formulated to assist ward teams to develop improvements in care practices.

Who maps which area?

Mapping has also raised issues of a personal nature for mappers around the area of relationships with other mappers and the mapping of their own areas. It was agreed very early that mappers would not map their own areas to avoid a conflict of interest. Only through honest and open communication within supervision sessions have some of these very difficult issues been resolved.

We consider that our training and development as a team has been fundamental to the growth of person-centred care practice as well as our knowledge and skills base. In response, a programme for annual in-house training has been developed. One team member is an advanced mapper and has facilitated a range of training events, including a programme to ensure inter-rater reliability. Formal links with mappers from another Trust have provided us with an opportunity to share our skills and developments in practice. There has also been an increased demand for presentations at local and national conferences. The team has had a key role to play at these conferences as we believe that sharing and networking are essential elements of person-centred care practice development.

The way forward

We acknowledge that significant advancements in the care of older people have been directly influenced by the implementation of a clear professional and practice strategy. The enthusiasm and commitment of clinical staff and mappers has also greatly influenced care practices.

At present we have implemented a person-centred care seminar programme for all clinical staff within the directorate which is facilitated by mappers. Future plans include an increased focus on the well-being of staff which will focus on a range of developments including more emphasis on clinical supervision in relation to positive person work in dementia care. The mappers are currently examining ways of introducing person-centred care practices with other client groups. There are plans to train more mappers from a range of backgrounds including other health care workers and informal carers.

Overall the experience for mappers and clinicians has been exciting and rewarding. Mappers feel that they have grown professionally and personally. Reflections from both mappers and clinical staff demonstrate the value of DCM to clients and staff alike.

References

Bradford Dementia Group (1997) *Evaluating Dementia Care: The DCM Method.* Seventh edition, University of Bradford.

Brooker D, Forster N, Banner A et al (1998) The efficacy of Dementia Care Mapping as an Audit Tool. Report of a 3 year British NHS evaluation. *Aging and Mental Health.* Volume 2 (1) 60-70.

Buckland S (1995) Dementia Care Mapping: Looking a Bit Deeper. *Signpost* 32 5-7.

Williams J & Rees J (1997). The use of Dementia Care Mapping as a method of evaluating care received by patients with dementia. *Journal of Advanced Nursing* 25 316-323.

• Published in *JDC*, July/Aug 2000.

11 Personal detractions – a personal account

DIANE BEAVIS & LIN JOHNSON

In 1995 four of the staff from Langbourne Ward attended a two-day course to become Dementia Care Mappers. Since this time DCM has been used as a means of evaluating the quality of life for the patients, and as a catalyst for change in the work environment.

AN EXAMINATION OF CARE PRACTICE IN THE LIGHT OF DCM REVEALING 'PERSONAL DETRACTIONS'

Langbourne is a continuing care assessment ward for people who have dementia. There is provision for respite and day care, plus emergency admissions when necessary. **1**

Personal Detractions

The Personal Detraction coding (PD) is used to record events which occur very briefly. At first glance they may seem somewhat trivial, but they can have severe, long lasting effects upon the person's sense of well-being.

PDs can range from minor discrepancies, such as being addressed by the wrong name, being slightly outpaced (talking or moving too fast for the person to keep up with), having sugar put in tea without being asked, to severe acts of mistreatment, eg 'frog marching' a client from one room to another against his will, intimidation, or being physically assaulted by a care worker. In each instance the acts are hurtful, and impair one's sense of well-being both psychologically and physically.

The list on the next page illustrates some of the common PDs which occur in a ward or long term care setting. It is provided by a nursing assistant who is qualified as a Dementia Care Mapper.

Consequences of personal detraction

All of the PDs mentioned, and many more which may occur less frequently, do damage to an individual's self-esteem and sense of well-being. This may result in the person becoming withdrawn, lethargic and unresponsive. Alternatively they may exhibit behavioural problems such as aggression, shouting or being un-cooperative. Ultimately this creates a vicious circle - the nursing staff feel stressed and are unable to manage the difficult behaviour. This results in care becoming depersonalized, causing the incidence of PDs to increase and further negative behaviour ensues.

It is this pattern of behaviour which is now being addressed by the staff on Langbourne ward. Following a discussion about the PDs mentioned in this article an action plan has been created (see next page).

The action plan illustrates the thought processes, feelings and behaviours which may occur when thoughtless or inappropriate care is given. It also outlines alternative options to creating a better atmosphere, whereby individuals feel respected and valued.

Conclusion

Personal Detractions may occur very briefly, but the damage they cause may be extremely detrimental to the individual's sense of well-being and self value.

It is easy to shrug off the comments illustrated in this article... 'they don't happen here...not while I am on duty'. This is the easy option, to ignore and accommodate such attitudes. However, if the philosophy of care is to improve the well-being of people with dementia, then we must stop and re-examine current practices and decide upon an overall strategy to improve relationships with the patients. This is not the easy option. It involves being honest with ourselves, acknowledging feelings, recognising distress both verbal and non-verbal, being able to interact in a supportive manner, being non-judgemental and valuing each person as a social being who has his/her own desires.

I think we have crossed the first barrier, we are being honest with ourselves, we have recognised and accepted that PDs do occur on our ward, and that this is not acceptable. The next step is to put our plan into action and see if we can change the care we give.

Changes will not happen overnight and we do not expect immediate results, but we have made a start.

• Published in *JDC*, July/Aug 1998.

1 Respite care provides short breaks for family carers.

Personal detraction	Thoughts, feelings and behaviour	Preventative action
1. Calling a person 'Sweetheart' or 'Good boy/girl'.	Thoughts: 'She can't remember my name.' 'I hate being called a good boy...I'm not a child,' Feelings: Isolated, lonely, unwanted, angry, resentful. Behaviour: Withdrawal, possible aggression.	Use preferred name and check with person (or relative) that this is acceptable. Apologise if accidentally mistaken for someone else.
2. Outpacing, eg walking too fast.	Thoughts: 'Why are they always in such a hurry?.. I can't go that fast.' Feelings: Overwhelmed, helpless, angry. Behaviour: Possible aggression, being obstinate, possible risk of falls due to walking too fast.	Slow down... check that you are not going too fast, do not pull, or walk backwards in front of person. Always walk at the person's side and go at his/her pace.
3. Talking over a person's head.	Thoughts: 'Please talk to me... I may not be able to answer, but I can hear you and I do understand.' Feelings: Neglect, abandonment, worthlessness, isolation. Behaviour: Withdrawal and possible depression. Shouting in an attempt to get attention.	Involve person in conversation: eg. if a colleague asks, 'Did you go to the market today?' you could answer, 'Yes, you used to enjoy going to the market didn't you Betty?' (patient's name). Direct conversation towards patient rather than back at colleague.
4. Taking away independence by doing self-care tasks without allowing the person to try for themselves.	Thoughts: 'I can do this... just let me do it on my own.' Feelings: Frustration, anger, annoyance, hopelessness. Behaviour: Aggression, shouting, 'difficult' behaviour, withdrawal and depression.	Check with person what he can do for himself and allow time and space to do so. Discreetly observe if necessary and prompt/intervene only when in obvious difficulty.
5. Saying, 'Yes, I will be back in a minute,' without any intention of doing so.	Thoughts: 'Who does she think she's fooling... she won't come back, they never do.' Feelings: Abandonment, worthlessness. Behaviour: Deterioration in physical abilities, eg. may become incontinent if not responded to immediately. May be at risk of accidental injury, if he tries to do something without assistance.	Avoid using this phrase. Answer truthfully ,eg: 'Tom, I'm sorry I can't help you at the moment, but I will ask another nurse to help you.' (Ensure that you do ask someone else.) Or say that you will help him as soon as you are able to do so.
6. A patient being told, 'If you don't hurry up, you won't get any more to eat/drink.'	Thoughts: 'I hate it here, it's like a prison... I wish I could go home.' Feelings: Loneliness, despair, worthlessness, anxious. Behaviour: Withdrawal and depression – possible aggression.	Staff to be made aware that this type of threat is not acceptable. Staff to provide a good role model, avoiding threats. Respond by saying, 'Don't worry Mr Rollings, there is plenty of time to eat your dinner, we'll put some pudding back for you.'

12 Putdowns and uplifts: signs of good or poor dementia care

DANIEL KUHN, JANE VERITY

In writing about a 'malignant social psychology' Tom Kitwood (1990, 1997a, 1997b; Kitwood & Bredin 1992) described a variety of ways in which the well-being of people with dementia could be undermined. His description of 17 'personal detractors' points out how they can be dehumanised by care staff and how awareness of such negative attitudes and behaviour could bring about change for the better. In this consciousness raising effort, Kitwood and Benson (1995) further contrasted the 'old culture' of dementia care characterised by command and control of persons with dementia with a 'new culture' marked by human respect and freedom. In this article, we build upon this work by describing a corresponding list of 17 ways in which personhood can be recognised and reinforced.

Based on extensive observations of people with dementia, we consider personal detractors or what we commonly refer to as 'putdowns' to be helpful in pointing out poor care practices. They indirectly point the way to a person-centred approach by bringing to awareness dehumanising behaviours of what not to do. There is, however, no systematic guide or clear framework for taking note of positive events that can help improve staff attitudes.

In order to enable care staff to embrace holistic care and positive values, an emphasis needs to be placed on identifying instances in which a person with dementia is uplifted by staff. In this way, staff can take pride in their efforts and better understand the impact of their work on the well-being of people in their care. Moreover, new staff can learn by good examples of individualised care and become acquainted with the values of the new culture of dementia care. Therefore, we propose a set of 'uplifts' that enrich the quality of life of people with dementia.

The language of personal detractors is intended to evoke an emotional response for the sake of changing attitudes. It is therefore negative, in some cases even harsh. Each of the 17 categories consists of a passive noun, emphasising their impersonal and chilling effects on persons with dementia. In contrast, we rely upon active verbs to describe ways that staff can make a positive difference in enhancing the life of people in their care. We will describe these contrasting terms and illustrate each one with case examples.

> THE 'NEW CULTURE' OF CARE ENABLES US TO IDENTIFY NEGATIVE SIGNS OF RELATING TO PEOPLE WITH DEMENTIA. WHAT OF THE POSITIVE ONES?

Treachery vs to be supportive

Treachery refers to forms of deception to distract, manipulate, or force someone into compliance. People with dementia will believe us if we tell them what they want to hear. They can often be deceived because of impaired memory and judgment. Treachery involves taking advantage of their cognitive deficits and overpowering them with our superior wits. Telling lies and 'therapeutic fibs' may make things go easier for staff but such deceptive practices undermine personhood. On the other hand, to be supportive of persons with dementia involves accepting their cognitive deficits as a disability yet viewing them as moral equals. This means we need to give full support to their views, their feelings and experiences – no matter how distorted or challenging these may seem. Their perceptions should be accepted.

A common scenario illustrates the difference between treachery and loyalty. A daughter has just left a care facility after a visiting her mother with dementia. Seeing that the resident is crying after the daughter's departure, a staff member attempts to 'reassure' her by saying, 'No need to feel upset. You daughter is just having a cup of tea – she'll be back in a short time.' Although well meaning, the statement is false and does not address the resident's emotional needs. Alternatively, the staff member might hug the resident and say in a caring tone of voice, 'I know you are upset when your daughter leaves. How about we take a walk together and then I make you a cup of tea?' This statement is intended to meet the resident's need for closeness and kindly redirects her to a pleasurable activity.

Disempowerment vs to empower

Disempowerment involves not allowing people with dementia to use their remaining abilities and failing to help them to complete actions that they have initiated. In contrast, in seeking to empower them, we actively look for ways to help them feel successful and put them back in control of their own lives.

For example, a staff member might handle all the steps of dressing a resident with dementia although the person is able to complete this task given time and encouragement. After all, it may be rationalised that it is necessary to overlook the resident's abilities in order to get the task of dressing done efficiently. In contrast, the resident's clothes might be laid out in proper sequence and the resident could be talked through each step of dressing and genuinely acknowledged for successfully completing the task. Although time consuming, this person-centred approach fosters well-being.

Infantilisation vs to honour

Infantilisation refers to treating people with dementia in a patronising or condescending manner, as an insensitive parent might treat a very young child. In contrast, to honour someone with dementia means honouring the essence of the human being, regarding each person as a complete individual with a unique personal history, and drawing on that person's strengths and resources instead of narrowly focusing on a current state of disability.

For instance, a staff member might disapprovingly remark after noticing a resident has become incontinent, 'Oh yuk! What a terrible smell you've made! Your incontinence pad needs changing right now.' In contrast, the same situation might be addressed compassionately with honour and regard if the staff member asks the resident, 'Anna, may I help you to your room to freshen up?'

Intimidation vs to empathise

Intimidation refers to inducing fear through threats, coercion, or physical power. In contrast, to empathise with people with dementia means to get at the root of their discomfort or resistance to care by addressing their needs first and foremost. It involves respecting their perspective by listening to underlying needs. The person's viewpoint is always considered, no matter how distorted it may appear.

For example, a staff member gives George his dentures but he refuses them. In response, the staff member might say, 'If you don't put them in your mouth, you will not get dinner today.' George may give in to this threat for fear of missing a meal, but he has been disrespected in the process and is reminded that he has little or no power in this place. On the other hand, a staff member might explore options with him by saying, 'George, is there something wrong with your dentures?' or 'Do you prefer to eat without your dentures today?'

Labelling vs to be descriptive

Labelling refers to using a category or word such as 'demented', 'wanderer', 'sundowner' etc as the basis for interacting with a person and for explaining behaviour. This involves putting the experience of people with dementia into boxes of our own making instead of describing their subjective experience. This tendency alienates us from their human-ness and instead turns them into lesser beings. To be descriptive, however, is to understand the complex nature of human behaviour and to use as many words as possible to describe the many facets of each person objectively. One diagnosis or label is not sufficient

to replace the name of a person with dementia, describe unmet needs or sum up an entire lifetime.

For example, referring to a person simply as 'a feeder' is dehumanising for all concerned. Describing this same person in terms of someone who can use utensils if assisted to do so focuses on the ability that is still intact and recognises the fact that this person would still prefer to eat unassisted. Or, instead of staff members announcing, 'Let's get the sundowners distracted before they start acting up' a more descriptive staff member might say, 'I can see that Sally, George, and Ida are getting a bit restless. Let's invite them to the lounge and sing some songs together.' Labels are a convenient and brief means of representing others and their experience. To be descriptive means to use as many words as necessary in order better understand the experience of others from their unique perspective.

Stigmatisation vs to affirm

Stigmatisation involves treating people as if they were diseased objects, aliens or outcasts. Rather than setting people with dementia apart for what they lack, to affirm is to recognise their humanity. In affirming the personhood of another, there is an effort to identify abilities and downplay disabilities. For example, John has advanced dementia and has been talking unintelligibly for the past 10 minutes. A staff member remarks to another, 'Don't bother with that one'. Pointing to her own head, she adds, 'There's nothing left up there.' Alternatively, a staff member might make eye contact with John and say, for example, 'John, you have an impish look in your eye. Tell me what's on your mind.'

Outpacing vs to pace

Outpacing is perhaps the most common putdown of all. It involves providing information or presenting choices at a rate too fast for a person to understand, or putting pressure on them to do things more rapidly than they can tolerate. In contrast, to pace is to recognise the slowed abilities of the person with dementia, each in their own way, and to adapt our speech and behaviour accordingly. This involves making necessary accommodations to the disabilities of people with dementia, in much the same way we might walk slowly alongside someone using crutches.

In a care setting, examples of outpacing are readily apparent to the trained eye. For instance, a staff member might say in a hurried voice to a resident, 'Ida, this morning the doctor is coming to see you. After lunch you are going to the hairdresser and tonight your son and daughter-in-law are picking you up for a family get together.' Ida becomes overwhelmed by all of this information given at once. She cannot retain it or understand it. Alternatively, the staff member could tell Ida one thing at a time and perhaps even write down this information to ensure that she has fully understood before taking the next step. Someone who keeps pace remembers that it is the responsibility of the sender to ensure the message is received.

Invalidation vs to validate

Invalidation refers to a failure to acknowledge the subjective reality of a person's experience, especially what they are feeling. In contrast, to validate people with dementia is to accept that their words, behaviour, and feelings are meaningful. Their confusion may require a careful eye or listening ear to figure out at times what they are attempting to convey. No matter how distorted their view of reality may appear to us, what they are experiencing is real to them.

For example, residents often declare after being admitted to a care facility, 'I want to go home.' An inexperienced staff member might reply, 'This is your home now' or 'You are at home' instead of addressing the resident's longing to feel loved, safe or comfortable. In another instance of invalidation, a resident says to a staff member, 'I'm hungry' and is told, 'You should not be hungry. You have just been fed.' Alternatively, a staff member might respect the need being expressed and reply, 'Can I bring you a snack of fruit or some biscuits?'

Banishment vs to include

Banishment involves sending a person away or excluding them physically or psychologically. To include someone means taking steps to reinforce membership in a group or social situation. It also means making allowances for behaviour that might otherwise be excluded and disapproved of and letting others know about this standard of inclusion.

For example, Fred repeatedly spits out his food at mealtimes while sitting with three other residents. In an exasperated state, a staff member removes Fred from the dining room and into his room without any more food. In contrast, Fred might be quietly asked to refrain from spitting or might be invited to join in eating with a staff member at another table.

Objectification vs to show recognition

Objectification is to treat a person like an object; there is no regard for feelings. For example, a staff member might suddenly push someone in a wheelchair without any prior explanation or permission. To show recognition means to treat the person in a respectful, dignified and personal manner. It is an affirmation of the person's humanity. In another instance, Sally is chatting with other residents when a staff member places a blood pressure cuff on her arm without any explanation. Conversation stops as the staff person goes about the task of taking Sally's blood pressure. Alternatively, the staff member could wait until Sally is back in her room, knocks on her door and ask, 'Sally, may I come in to take your blood pressure?'

Ignoring vs to acknowledge

Ignoring refers to situations in which staff members carry on a conversation or activity as if the person with dementia is not present. On the other hand, to acknowledge someone with dementia is to keep in mind that the person deserves to be acknowledged. For example, staff members talking with each other while assisting residents with eating is a common example of this type of putdown. Alternatively, staff members put aside their need to talk with each other until a better time. They put their whole focus and attention on the residents, enabling them to have a positive social experience while eating their meal.

Imposition vs to promote autonomy

Imposition refers to forcing a person to do something, overriding their desire or denying the possibility of personal choice. On the other hand, promoting autonomy involves recognising personal preferences and offering choices, no matter how small. For example, Virginia is helped to put on a grey dress without any consultation. Alternatively, a staff member might pick out two of Virginia's favorite dresses and while showing her both choices say, 'Today will it be the blue dress or the orange one?' In this scenario, the number of choices has been narrowed to an understandable level and Virginia can express her preference without a problem.

Withholding vs to be compassionate

Withholding involves refusing to give attention that is requested or to meet an evident need. In contrast, to be compassionate is to simply to give from the heart, to wish to enrich the other person's life and give attention to their needs. For example, Harriet is sitting in a wheelchair and crying out, 'Help me! Help me! Help me!' It is obvious that she is in distress. A staff member declares, 'There she goes again with her attention-seeking behaviour.' Although similar to ignoring, withholding is a more active type of putdown in that the person's presence is acknowledged yet a need for help is not addressed. Alternatively, a staff member might instead greet Harriet warmly, give her a hug and in a caring, loving voice say, 'How can I help you, Harriet?'

Accusation vs to understand

Accusation refers to blaming a person for actions or failures of actions that arise from lack of ability. This is often the result of lack of understanding about the reasons underlying the behaviour. On the other hand, to understand means to recognise that there usually is a reasonable explanation for the behaviour. For example, Stanley is found taking some items from another resident's room and a staff member says, 'You are stealing again. Put those things down. They don't belong to you!' Alternatively, a staff member understands there is a reason for this behaviour, explores with Stanley what he has been looking for, and works on meeting this need in another way.

Disruption vs to stand back

Disruption is suddenly intruding upon or interrupting a person's thought or behaviour. In such instances, staff members put their own agenda ahead of the needs of the person with dementia. However, to stand back is to look at what is happening within the person's current frame of reference and to wait for a good time to intervene. For example, several residents including Betty are enjoying a singing group when a staff member walks into the middle and loudly declares, 'I have not yet bathed Betty... Betty come with me.' On the other hand, the staff member could wait until the group activity has ended and then discreetly asks, 'Are you ready for a warm bath now, Betty?'

Mockery vs to pay respect

Mockery is perhaps the most troubling behaviour to witness firsthand and fortunately it is rarely seen among staff. For example, Elizabeth repetitively makes the sound, 'Ooh! Ooh! Ooh!' In response, a staff member mimics Elizabeth, yells out, 'You sound like a damn foghorn!'and laughs loudly. In contrast, to pay respect involves recognising that a person's impairments do not represent the whole self. Each person is worthy of respect regardless of their capacity or incapacity. Thus, instead of making a hurtful remark, the staff member attempts to understand Elizabeth's mood.

Disparagement vs to boost self-esteem

Disparagement is telling a person that they are incompetent, useless or worthless by giving them messages that are damaging to their self-esteem. On the other hand, to boost self-esteem is to be sensitive to the things the person with dementia offers to help with, and then find ways to do them successfully. Thus, to recognise each effort will lead to more effort whereas disparaging effort will likely ensure that further effort will not take place. The success of an effort is not measured by the outcome but through appreciation for

the process. For example, Mary offers to set the table but is told, 'No, you sit down. You are retired now so we take care of you.' In contrast, staff might say, 'Thank you, Mary! I would love your help. Could you start by folding these napkins?'

Summary

Dementia has traditionally been described in terms of irreversible loss of brain cells leading to deterioration, disability, and death. This pessimistic view stands in stark contrast to Kitwood who envisioned that personhood could be maintained and enhanced until the end of life through what he termed 'positive person work' (1997, p89). This refers to a host of rich interactions between staff and persons with dementia. Good care practices need to be identified, appreciated, taught, and replicated if persons with dementia are to be freed from the myths and mistakes of the old culture of care. Such optimistic work is central to transforming the culture of care and promoting lifelong vitality.

• Published in *JDC*, Sept/Oct 2002.

References

Bradford Dementia Group (1997) *Evaluating Dementia Care: The DCM Method*, 7th ed. Bradford Dementia Group, University of Bradford.

Kitwood T (1997) *Dementia Reconsidered: The Person Comes First.* Open University Press, Buckingham.

Kitwood T (1990) The dialectics of dementia with particular reference to Alzheimer's disease. *Ageing and Society* 1990; 10: 177-196.

Kitwood T & Bredin K (1992) *Person to Person: A Guide to the Care of Those with Failing Mental Powers*. Gale Centre Publications, Loughton.

Kitwood T & Benson S (eds 1995) *The New Culture of Dementia Care*. Hawker Publications, London.

13 Haloperidol, hips and toenails...

TRACY PACKER, MICHELLE JEFFERIES

Mrs T arrived on our ward one summer day from a medical ward in the main hospital. She had been sent to await her place for admission to a local 'EMI' Unit. [1]

The ambulance crew came and went, leaving behind an elderly lady who was very agitated and distressed. Clearly frightened, she took a long time to respond in any other way, to either the staff or patients on the ward.

This transfer may have been a routine event for the team working there, but for Mrs T the implications were huge. At the age of 83, she had spent no less than four months in three different wards, recovering after an operation to repair her fractured hip. Yet again she was faced with the arduous task of trying to remember the routine, the people, the layout and all the many other details which hospital staff take for granted.

The nurse on the previous ward had passed on some information about Mrs T, describing her as a lady with vascular dementia who was not compliant with her daily care needs. She consistently refused help, including toileting, daily hygiene needs and dressing assistance. She had developed a urinary tract infection and constipation, and was doubly incontinent. This had not been a problem before her admission to hospital. Her legs were swollen and painful, and she had been immobile for the most part since her hip operation.

She was prescribed haloperidol five times a day, with chloral hydrate at night in order to try and calm her down. This was not working.

Following a change in their admission criteria and role within the hospital, the team receiving Mrs T had only just begun to admit people with a dementing illness. Many of the staff were apprehensive, feeling de-skilled and lacking in knowledge about the care of this client group. Mrs T's responses to their care only seemed to reinforce those concerns; for many she represented their worst fears about working with people with dementia.

After a day or two Mrs T's continued non-compliance, and aggressive responses when receiving most care including feeding, began to cause staff considerable concern - not

> WHEN MRS T WAS TAKEN OFF HER 'CALMING' MEDICATION, SHE EMERGED AS A PERSON AND STAFF COULD BEGIN A PROCESS OF DISCOVERY

least because of the invariable screaming, kicking, scratching and biting which accompanied even the most minimal contact, and which was distressing for everyone involved or within earshot.

When her personal care needs were finally met, Mrs T would make an attempt to get around without using the walking frame provided. She had now begun to 'furniture walk', teetering precariously between unstable chairs and tables, before sitting down on the nearest bed and folding other patients' clothes or 'tidying' their cupboards.

As these people did not have dementia and could not understand her behaviour, they would often get angry with her or the nursing staff, who continually had to 'take her away' and lead her back to her own bed area. This only increased Mrs T's determination to try again, which caused even greater frustration within the unit.

Highly demanding

At night time, despite regular doses of haloperidol and chloral hydrate, Mrs T became even more active and demanding of nurses' time. If she needed the toilet she would refuse to use the commode provided and urinate on the floor nearby. Sometimes she would even urinate on a nearby bed. She would frequently call out or attempt to leave her bed, as if she was afraid of being on her own in the dark.

The staff were concerned that she might fall and hurt herself, and had placed cotsides on the bed to try and reduce this risk. But this had made matters worse, as Mrs T would then try and climb over the top of them, or slide down the bed to get out at the bottom. This only increased the risk of a more damaging fall, or bruising and cuts on her delicate skin. Other tired and anxious patients were getting more and more irritable with her.

Things were getting worse and worse. Mrs T's daughter (her only visitor) had become reluctant to come in and see her because she felt her visits only made her mother even more distressed.

During the staff handovers in those first 10 days, Mrs T's responses were discussed in detail. It was agreed that

---

[1] EMI stands for Elderly Mentally Infirm. In the UK some nursing homes are registered as 'EMI' to care for people with dementia.

events could not continue in this way. The team agreed that key nurses needed to work with her at all times to build up a trusting relationship. Their main aims at this time were to maintain her safety while she was improving her skills at getting around, promote her independence as much as possible, and try to alleviate her anxieties about contact with staff during direct personal care.

During these discussions the team concluded that Mrs T was highly independent and very sensitive about exposing any part of her body to other people, particularly during intimate personal care. She would not allow anyone to wash or dress her, and it was realised that she did not have any of her own clothes. She hated continence pads and refused to wear them, pulling them out and throwing them disdainfully on the floor or ripping them to shreds.

The team thought it was ironic that in her assessment on the previous ward the categories 'Expressing sexuality', and 'Self-esteem and dignity' had 'Vascular dementia' written next to them. It was as if Mrs T could not be expected to have any self-esteem, dignity or sexual expression because she had dementia.

Mrs T's relationship with her daughter had also been severely restricted, and we felt this important link needed to be re-established. Staff began to contact the daughter regularly to keep her updated, and she was persuaded to bring some personal items of clothing in for her mother. We also discussed the use of cotsides and she consented to their removal, agreeing that the risks outweighed the benefits. She was also persuaded to bring in fruit and other 'finger' foodstuffs to tempt Mrs T, who still refused to be fed at any time.

The situation appeared to relax for a day or two, until one morning after a distressing night, an episode of incontinence in her bed and yet another confrontational bedside wash, a tepid breakfast was thrown in disgust at the nurse trying to feed her. Then she kicked in the face the chiropodist who was trying to treat her feet.

By this time the team had called for some advice from a specialist dementia care nurse, who was undertaking some Dementia Care Mapping (DCM) on the unit that day. Mrs T was just one of the people being observed, but in this instance the 'map' was abandoned and Mrs T's care was discussed immediately. The member of trained staff learning about DCM was encouraged to think about and interpret what she saw.

Careful observation

Mrs T's fierce independence, her distress, her marked hand tremor (which had not previously been noted), and the 'guarding' (protecting) of her hip had all been observed during the DCM. We thought it very likely that the tremor was a side effect of haloperidol. If the tremor could be stopped, Mrs T would be able to hold cutlery and feed herself, assist in her washing and dressing, and use her walking frame. As it was, she could not even lift a small cup of tea to her lips without spilling the contents.

It also became clear she was experiencing pain in the hip which had been operated upon - and it was this side which the chiropodist had been attempting to treat.

The doctor was called to the ward, and the nurse in charge explained the situation. The haloperidol was stopped immediately, and suitable pain killers prescribed. These were given to Mrs T straight away. Other factors surrounding her care were discussed with the dementia nurse – for example the importance of finding out more about Mrs T's life before her hospital admission, and the need for nurses to give her social contact and attention at times other than during care tasks, in order to help re-build her confidence in them.

The following morning, much to the amazement of the ward team (most of whom had been rather cynical about the withdrawal of haloperidol) Mrs T got out of bed, walked with her frame to the toilet, washed herself, dressed and ate a full breakfast. She was much more relaxed and even smiling at times. The tremor was still noticeable, but had significantly reduced.

Over the course of the next few weeks the team found out more about Mrs T, which helped explain much of her behaviour. For many years after her husband died she had lived on her own, refusing social services involvement of any kind, and never leaving the house alone. She had been, by her own admission at that time, phobic about being institutionalised. She had felt this way for over 30 years, although a reason for this fear was never fully established.

Through a stroke of luck we discovered that Mrs T had worked as head of the laundry at the local homeopathic hospital for 30 years. She recognised a nurse who used to work there, who recalled that Mrs T was very efficient at her job. This explained her preoccupation with other people's clothing. Once this was understood, Mrs T spent many industrious moments folding newly laundered bed linen for the staff, and sorting out piles of hospital nightwear.

Mrs T was also very particular about toilet seats. She would use a 'proper' toilet, but even then would never sit down properly on the seat, no matter how clean it was. She would squat on her haunches and 'hover' above the seat to use the toilet. Through trial and error staff learned that any attempt to make her sit on it properly would result in anger and distress. It was important that any new or temporary staff were told of this, rather than learning the hard way.

Mrs T would not sit on a commode under any circumstances, so it was removed and no further attempts were made to make her use it. Once her mobility began to improve, the inappropriate urinating ceased as long as she was able to use the main toilet.

Mrs T would also leave the toilet cubicle 'mid-stream' if the member of staff left the area to give her the privacy that is normally valued. She would only complete her toileting needs if the staff member stayed in the cubicle with her, or talked to her continuously from outside the door. Either way, they could not go away even for a short time, or Mrs T would leave the cubicle partially undressed in a panic to find them.

This behaviour baffled the team, and no convincing explanation was ever found. Was she afraid of falling into the toilet? Had something nasty happened to her in a small enclosed space? What had happened that left her so terrified of being on her own? We never did find out, but at least a satisfactory compromise had been reached.

Mrs T's night time sleeping pattern never really changed, and she would still wander about looking for company or something to do. If this need was addressed, she would generally be quite quiet. If she had been able to use the toilet, she would sleep for four to six hours, which seemed to be enough for her. The team realised that if they pulled three of the four bedside curtains around her, rather like a small room, she treated that area as her own space.

Special attention

At about three thirty in the afternoon, the noise of the children in the crèche behind the hospital would make her agitated. She would talk about her need to take her children safely home from school. This maternal need was identified, and some members of the team took extra time to be with her during this part of the day, to talk about her love of children. Alternatively, she could often be seen walking arm in arm with a nurse who would be getting on with tasks that only need one arm free! Otherwise she would sit in the staff office and chat with the nurses while they completed administrative tasks.

It was discovered that she loved teddy bears, and took ownership of any stray soft toys that were left behind. One in particular stayed at her bedside at all times, and was a great source of comfort. She increasingly sought tactile contact with staff, most of whom responded well to this although some found this aspect of her personality more challenging. Often she would spontaneously hug a person and then ask them to sit on her knee! This became a common sight.

Despite our efforts, Mrs T hated the shift changeover, as this meant her nurse for the day would go home. As a way of dealing with this, she would mask her worries in a joke. Her parting words to that person would be, "I'll throw you out of the window I will" Perhaps this too arose from her need to have some control over the daily comings and goings.

Throughout this period, the team maintained regular phone contact with Mrs T's daughter, who was only too pleased to answer questions and receive updates about her mother's progress. We explained that her mother was now very affectionate, getting upset even when members of staff went home, and that we saw this as an understandable reaction probably indicating her need for stability. We reported that the distress was short lived, and now that staff knew more about Mrs T, less difficult to allay.

Towards the end of Mrs T's admission her daughter was eventually persuaded to come in and stay for longer visits, bringing with her chocolates and sweets. Mrs T was at her happiest and most relaxed at these times.

In November, Mrs T and her teddy bear were successfully placed in a nursing home. The information exchanged outlined all of her known foibles. No one wanted either Mrs T, her daughter, or other care staff to experience the trauma of learning the hard way, as they had done. The only thing the staff had not been able to do by this time, was to cut her toenails' – not surprising perhaps after the episode with the chiropodist.

Four weeks later, just before Christmas, staff from the ward visited Mrs T in her new home to give her a Christmas present. They were overwhelmed with her progress. A well dressed, smiling Mrs T proudly showed them her bathroom, the photographs of her husband on their wedding day, (she would never discuss him in hospital), and at long last, her newly cut toenails.

• Published in *JDC*, Nov/Dec 1997.

14 Facing up to the Bills

TRACY PACKER

Somehow, we have to find a way to underpin care work with a person-centred philosophy, even when environments and resources fall far short of necessary standards.

We should not, I would argue, put person-centred care 'on hold' until some indeterminate moment in time when things might be different. On the contrary, every little bit counts. Small ripples can make big waves, but only if large numbers of those involved in direct clinical care are prepared to be proactive in spite of these limitations, and accept the psychological conflict this will involve. For this reason team leaders and the organisations that they work in must look more closely at the psychological costs to care workers caught up in this conundrum and, in the meantime, consider ways to minimise them.

Here I offer an opportunity to consider what is being demanded of care workers within a person-centred philosophy when they are routinely expected to spend time with someone who may make alarming demands on their personal resources.

What can you do?

[There's] a particular patient, his mind is on the go but you can't actually get him to do anything. He can't channel... it's all over the place, it's haywire. He wants to do something, he's frustrated and angry. He wants something but there's nothing. What can you give him to occupy him – WHAT? You can't even sit down and talk to him to occupy him. You can NOT entertain the man, there's nothing you can do.

This quotation was taken from my own transcripts of recorded interviews with a range of staff who were involved in the medical care of people with dementia in hospital (Packer 1999). Although this conversation took place almost five years ago, I can still vividly remember how the staff member used her hands to emphasise her words and illustrate her feeling of intense frustration, even anger. She was keen and enthusiastic, willing to try anything if it might make a difference, but on this day, she felt that she had exhausted all her options. Her feeling of disempowerment was tangible, and it stayed with me long after she left the room. I wondered if her patient had recognised it as well.

I knew the man to whom she was referring. Bill (not his

> **CARE WORKERS WHO WANT TO WORK IN A PERSON-CENTRED WAY WITH LIMITED RESOURCES FACE PSYCHOLOGICAL CONFLICT**

real name) had had a responsible and supervisory 'foreman' role in his work, and had also been a semi-professional footballer. He loved being with his wife (who came in to see him every day for a couple of hours) and meal times. However, he disliked crowds, patronising conversation or tasks, and anybody who invaded his body space. His limited speech revolved around a number of very expressive swear words, but even this ability was disappearing fast. He had been walking. although unsteadily, when he first arrived at the unit, but had become wheelchair dependent, despite great efforts to keep him moving. He was doubly incontinent, and unable to wash and dress himself. He had been given a diagnosis of probable Lewy body dementia.

It did not take a genius to work out just how disempowered Bill was feeling as a result of what the dementing process was doing so rapidly to his mind, his body and his most significant remaining relationship – the one with his wife. During his admission, many members of staff were kicked, punched, and bitten despite their best efforts to develop some kind of a relationship with him. Bill did not appear to trust anyone and at one point had successfully created his own 'exclusion zone' that extended just beyond arms reach around him. Anyone entering this zone had to abide by complex rules of engagement if they were to emerge unscathed. Unfortunately other patients occasionally strayed into the zone, and if quick acting staff were not at hand, the consequences could be very distressing. The anxiety that this caused to everyone on the unit and their visitors was immense. It appeared that Bill was in some way seizing control from those around him, and reasserting himself (in keeping with his former role as a foreman), so that he could retain control over a very visible aspect of his daily life. The more disempowered he felt, the more control he needed to impose on those who surrounded him.

Cycle of breakdown

Unfortunately this became a destructive cycle. The more Bill imposed himself on care workers in this way, the more they withdrew from him. This was entirely understandable, but it meant that most care workers only had contact with him when absolutely necessary, usually when unpleasant physical care needed to be undertaken. These tasks would be efficiently completed, usually with two care workers: one to hold flailing limbs, while the other completed the task. This simply reinforced their perception of Bill as an aggressive man, and his perception of them as agents of control. Both parties had concluded that every encounter with the other was destined to be an antagonistic one, and their particular defence mechanisms became more deeply entrenched.

Ironically, if Bill picked up any element of fear or uncertainty in those who worked with him, he became worse. We were never quite sure whether this was because he felt insecure and vulnerable if not absolutely convinced of a care worker's confidence in what they were doing, or whether there was an element of psychological bullying (feeding his need to feel in control).

Whatever the case, these particular coping mechanisms were already being used long before Bill's admission to the unit, and to some degree had been inadvertently reinforced after his arrival.

As a result, it was to be a long time before any degree of trusting relationship between staff and patient was to develop. It was to take even longer to unpick and replace the coping mechanisms of both parties with more sensitive responses. In the meantime, no nursing home in the area (not even 'EMI' homes) was prepared to take Bill on as his needs were described as 'far too complex... could not be met in this environment'. Whether they liked it or not, Bill and the team somehow had to find a mutually acceptable way of living alongside each other.

The situation seemed to deteriorate when, after much debate and discussion, a number of staff members felt that they had to withdraw from involvement with his direct physical care, or any non-emergency contact. Many staff had been on the receiving end of his teeth, fists and feet on a daily basis and could not cope with the strain this was putting them under. Some were simply frightened and felt that he knew this. While the team as a whole respected the need to support colleagues under this kind of stress, the outright refusal of some to take part in any direct aspect of his physical care came as a shock. Managers could agree or disagree with this perspective, nevertheless, the understandable feeling was:

'Dementia or not, nobody should have to be on the receiving end of such violence in their day to day work. We should be paid danger money for this!'

Fortunately enough people were prepared to continue to try to work with him, but as their numbers dwindled, the same individuals were having to deal with increasing levels of stress on an ongoing basis. The inequality of this was beginning to take its toll, and increasingly polarised views about the approach to be taken began to lead to fragmentation of the team.

As if this wasn't enough, another key aspect of Bill's daily life resulted in further anxiety – for him as well as the staff. For about six months before he became completely wheel-chair dependent, Bill could not stand up straight for more than a second without falling over. His limb co-ordination and spatial awareness seemed to be completely out of kilter, yet he seemed to have no insight about this. His wish to be engaged and involved, coupled with his need to feel in control, meant that he spent the whole day rocking forward in his chair and hauling himself to a semi-standing position. Most of the time he inevitably fell back heavily into his chair, but on odd and unpredictable occasions he would lurch forward. Usually, a member of staff nearby would launch themselves over to catch him just before he fell, risking back injury and, more often than not, a well-aimed thump. On one or two occasions there would be nobody near, and he would fall onto his face with a sickening thud.

Bill always seemed to be covered in bruises, and it was miraculous that he had not sustained more serious injuries. This led to tremendous tension among staff who were embarrassed by both bruises and the endless accident forms and phonecalls to his wife. He would not tolerate a head or hip guard, hit out at anyone who approached him in an attempt to redirect his attention to something else, and could not tolerate even minimal sedation (he was hypersensitive to it).

The team was aware that the use of physical restraint was very controversial, and in any case believed it would cause him even greater distress and lead to increased anger. However, at moments when they had reached the end of their tether, or could not provide the close supervision necessary, they would resort to putting a table in front of him. As a restraint this was generally ineffective because he would often push it over and get up anyway, but this at least gave the staff a warning and usually enough time to get to him before he fell.

Bill was a man who could not bear being surrounded by many people, and hated loud noises, but he equally hated to be alone and was less easy to supervise discreetly in his own room. He couldn't bear group activities, and on the occasions he took part, he spent the time swearing loudly and making offensive personal comments about the staff and other patients. Once the team had registered this, he often sat apart from the immediate activity, but with a vantage-point that allowed him to survey what was going on without taking direct part in it. This was a good idea in itself, but ironically a care mapping exercise identified that his regular seating position was right under one of the ward phones. This was easily and quickly remedied, and telephone-related assaults dropped dramatically!

Feeding self-esteem

Most of the time other patients and their relatives avoided Bill. Many voiced their fear explicitly. Those staff who felt able to do so, however, continued to attempt a more personal one-to-one approach with him. They knew it was possible if he felt safe enough and trusted the person concerned, because there were times that he would allow his wife to sit, hold his hand and briefly kiss him. There were admittedly times when he would not allow it and this distressed his wife, but at least the team recognised that it was not impossible for him to accept such contact. Bill clearly enjoyed mealtimes, and appeared at his most calm and relaxed on occasions when he was being discreetly assisted to eat. With time, the team learned that he gained even greater satisfaction when presented with food he could pick up with his fingers and feed to himself. Empowering him in this important and public aspect of daily living was a huge step forward, and being able to share this new knowledge with his wife meant that she too could bring in food that he could eat in this way. This enriched their relationship and reinforced her continuing role in his care.

The results of staff efforts during non-food related activities were variable. At worst, these attempts would result in a cup of coffee, a punch or a kick being thrown at the staff member. At best, Bill would very occasionally let someone hold his hand and sit quietly beside him. Most of the occasions in between, Bill could be seen to grasp both chair arms and draw himself as far back into his seat as possible. He would then start to grind his teeth. If engagement by the staff member had not been obviously successful at this point, he would then inhale sharply, as if raising himself to his full sitting height, stretch his head back and stare fixedly down his nose at the person in front of him. Initially this was always interpreted as an aggressive posture and usually succeeded in making anybody nearby back off immediately – if they didn't, this posture was almost always followed with a flailing limb.

We could not establish a pattern to this response. Staff who had previously been successful would be just as likely to receive this response as those who had not. Gender, ethnicity, uniform colour and communication style did not seem to be consistent predictors. It was thought that these actions might be an indication of pain, but regular analgesia did not allay these non-verbal messages. Looking back, I believe this was in fact a defensive posture rather than offensive, borne out of intense fear of something we could not understand. It is possible that he could have been hallucinating, although we could never really tell.

Over time, the staff began to evolve a way of supervising Bill without necessarily 'special-ing' him on an explicitly one-to-one basis as it was having inconsistent results. It was also putting tremendous pressure on staff who really did not know how to relate to him, and generally found the experience quite unpleasant. This approach involved agreeing that one person would remain in the communal area of the ward, in order to keep him within discreet visual range at all times. This strategy seemed an obvious one, but it invariably meant that everybody else on duty had to work physically harder and more efficiently elsewhere on the unit because of the 'loss' of that member of the team. It

was ironic that sometimes the person 'on watch' in the communal area would be viewed as having an easy time, when even indirect supervision of this kind took its toll on some care workers who were in a state of perpetual anxiety about this role.

DCM exercises illustrated that the sole member of staff in the communal area did not only have Bill to worry about, but often had the safety of numerous individuals to maintain. On many occasions, mappers would have to suspend the observation process temporarily and help out. It appeared that far too much was being expected of that one individual. This was supported by the common perception that it wouldn't look good with departments outside the unit if Bill actually fell while staff were supposed to be watching him. In fairness, given the number of accident forms being completed, there was probably an element of truth in this. Those staff brave enough to take on this role in the communal area appeared to be in a no win situation, and a mutiny was brewing once again.

A change in approach

The team changed tactics. Rather than having the same member of staff in the communal area for long periods of time, the whole team began to relieve that person at natural points in their own work pattern. For instance, if one member of staff had finished assisting a patient and they had wished to go to the communal area, that staff member would go with them and spend a little time helping them to locate a suitable chair and get settled in. The staff member already there could then request additional help if it was needed for anything, or arrange to leave the area to do something else. This more informal rotation system meant that everybody experienced what it felt like to be there alone, and was more inclined to help out whenever possible. It also meant that no one had to tolerate excessively long periods under pressure, and the team became adept at recognising each other's symptoms of stress – sometimes even the indicators of increased patient ill-being in the communal atmosphere.

They were certainly making significant progress, but in reality the team never really found an entirely acceptable strategy of supervision and engagement that worked well for both them and Bill at the same time. In the end nature took its course, and gradually provided a solution to the question of his immediate safety. After about six months of this dilemma, Bill appeared to lose all remaining limb co-ordination and balance, and lost interest in trying to stand up. By this time, he had developed a good relationship with a small number of staff members who had developed complex strategies for assessing his mood, initiating contact and recognising when the optimum time for contact was over! After several detailed planning meetings, a nursing home did eventually accept him. Just before lunchtime, a member of staff armed herself with a detailed plan of care and accompanied him there. She remained

Just one of those days? Perspectives on conflict in care

09:25 Everything had been fine when Albert woke up and the lady with the friendly face had helped him get washed and dressed. This was a blessed relief, because he could not understand how his cardigan fitted around his arms. He knew it did – he could tell he'd worn it before, but it was a bit of a puzzle. The friendly lady had disappeared now, he didn't know who she was exactly but she'd helped him before and he felt he could trust her. He wasn't sure about this place and he missed his wife, but breakfast had been good. He wondered what would happen next?

09:30 Sally was exhausted already and she'd only got three people up since she'd come on duty at 7am. The clock hands seemed to move faster the more behind she became. Molly and Beatrice would have to be 'done' next as they both needed two people to help them, but Dave was going to be caught up at the other end for the next 20 minutes. This would be a good time to have a cup of tea, thought Sally with relief – just for once I might actually get my full break. As she left, she could see Albert out of the corner of her eye. 'All right Albert?' she said smiling at him as she walked by. Thank goodness she'd got him out of the way early on in the shift.

09:35 There was no one else at the table now, everyone else seemed to know where to go. Albert wondered what he had to do next, then the smiling lady had asked him if he was 'All right' as she walked by. His tentative reply dissolved in a draught of air as she left. 'Not really... What do I do now?'

09:40 Esther the housekeeper noticed the new chap sitting alone at the table. 'Aww, bless him,' she thought to herself. 'All right?' she shouted cheerfully as she busied herself past him.

09:45 Dave was running late. He had promised to help Sally with her two ladies, and she was due back in five minutes. Bernard however, had been in a foul mood, and had taken it out on him this morning, so things had taken much longer than usual. Dave had finally developed some kind of a rapport, when Albert the new bloke had walked into the room asking what he should do next. Bernard of course, had been less than polite, and to avert a showdown, Dave had walked Albert back to the table he'd been sat at earlier. 'Just sit there a minute, Sally will be back soon – all right?' said Dave firmly, as he wondered how long it would take to pacify Bernard after this.

09:50 Albert couldn't believe it, he'd tried to find someone who could tell him what the plan was, when a complete stranger had shouted abuse at him. Then another chap had practically hustled him away as if it was his fault! Well perhaps not exactly hustled, but why did he feel as if he'd done something wrong? Albert thought he'd better try and find someone else to help him out. Now then, where was that friendly lady?

09:55 Sally had arrived back on the unit to the sound of Molly shouting. 'Go away. I said GO AWAY! I don't know what you've got to do – How should I know? Help! Help!' Sally hurried to Molly's bedside. Albert, who was protesting his innocence, looked very upset and Molly was furious. Sally took a deep breath. 'All right Molly, everything will be fine, Albert isn't going to hurt you.' She turned to Albert and offered her arm 'Come on Albert – come with me, let's sit you down and have a nice cup of tea.' As she walked over to Albert and put his tea on the table, Sally hoped that Dave would be ready to help her with Molly who was now in quite a state. 'There you are Albert, hot and sweet as you like it... all right?' She didn't see the look on his face as she turned and walked hurriedly away.

10:05 Things were going from bad to worse. Albert felt completely 'at sea' propelled by forces he couldn't control. He sensed that there wasn't a plan after all, and this made him feel very uncomfortable. The best thing he could do was leave. The only problem was – how to find the way out?

10:15 Dave couldn't believe how the morning was turning out. There he was carrying clothes, towels, toiletries and other associated paraphernalia when Albert stopped him again. He really was getting quite agitated. 'Esther,' he yelled, before Albert could speak, 'can you make Albert a cup of tea?' Esther appeared looking a little harassed. 'Go with Esther, Albert, she'll make you a nice cup of tea... all right?'

10:25 Marion had been caught up with phone calls and administration all morning and had just met the chap who had come in yesterday. She couldn't believe how aggressive he was. 'I only asked him if he was all right....he didn't have to bite my head off! I know,' she thought, 'I'll make him a nice cup of tea, that should calm him down.'

10:35 Sally and Dave looked up in alarm at the sound of raised voices, breaking china, and swearing from the other room. Promising Molly they would return 'in a minute', they both rushed to see what on earth was going on. Marion, looking pale and a little shocked, appeared to be wearing the contents of the teacup down her front. Albert, puce with rage had turned to them both and shouted, 'I DON'T WANT ANOTHER BLOODY CUP OF TEA – I JUST WANT TO GO HOME!'

Sally and Dave turned simultaneously to each other 'It's just one of THOSE days,' they both thought, raising their eyes to the sky. 'These days, they seem to happen all the time!'

with him during lunch, working alongside the staff at the home until he went to bed that evening. The discharge was successful, and he stayed there until his death two and a half years later.

Long-term lessons

It is easy to look back at a situation and consider what we might have done instead, but Bill taught us a lesson that has taken me several years to understand more fully. Bill and the team all just muddled along together, relying on good will, a degree of bloody-mindedness, and a little bit of luck. No plan as such was ever formulated. One evolved as each mistake was made, and those concerned tried to find ways of not doing the same thing again.

A regular, structured review of the situation happened rarely if ever. Staff did not always feel they could safely express their true feelings about how it felt to be on the receiving end and occasionally resorted to disaffected huddles in linen cupboards. We did not know where to begin, and were only developing strategies in response to the situation as it unfolded before us. Until then, anticipatory planning was not a familiar concept to the team, and every mistake felt like a major setback. There have been several other 'Bills' since then, and each time we have learned a little more. Everyone in the field probably has their own 'Bill', and may feel that they 'failed' these individuals. However, if we can learn from what they have taught us, then we have not completely failed after all.

The informal rotation system in the communal area has stayed in place. It doesn't always work, and occasionally realisation dawns that no one is 'down there'. Currently the team, who work in a predominantly 'medicalised' context, are wrestling with the concept of developing occupational and creative skills, and using these while they are in the communal area. However, this is a huge and challenging step, and we have some way to go. Despite this, what I admire most about my colleagues, is their guts and determination to keep trying, often with people with dementia whom everyone else has given up on. We have a long way to go before we can say that truly person-centred care is taking place on this unit but, my goodness, they are giving it their best shot.

• Published in *JDC*, July/Aug 2000.

References

Packer T (1999) Attitudes Towards Dementia Care: The Role of Education and Morale in Health Care Teams, in Adams T & Clarke CL (eds) *Dementia Care: Developing Partnerships in Practice.* Bailliere Tindall.

Packer T (2000) Does person-centred care exist? *Journal of Dementia Care* 8(3) 19-21.

15 Is it really such a risk?

CAROLINE BAKER

'We couldn't possibly do that' comes the reply – again. You may think I am asking people to jump into a turbulent river or walk across the road blindfolded. No, I am merely asking that the person with dementia be included in everyday activities.

> **WHY ARE RESIDENTS SOMETIMES 'PROTECTED' TOO MUCH FROM ACTIVITIES THAT COULD BENEFIT THEM?**

While carrying out training sessions with care staff, I talk to them about empowering the person with dementia, engaging them in activity that is meaningful to them. All too often, when I am carrying out DCM (Bradford Dementia Group 1997), I see people being totally disempowered and prevented from carrying out tasks that in reality pose no real risk. So why do we continue to disempower people?

Until a few months ago, I worked for ExtraCare Charitable Trust, a company that fostered a belief of 'fun first, fear later'. Nothing was impossible if you employed the knowledge and expertise of others to facilitate the activity safely. Having taken people with dementia rock climbing, abseiling, horse riding and canoeing and seeing the high levels of well-being they experienced, I am now finding it difficult to come back to 'grass roots' with my feet firmly on the ground.

Obviously, we all have to be aware of the possibility of litigation; we need to carry out risk assessments, observe health and safety policies and infection control policies. But who are we protecting – them or us? For our own satisfaction and creative self-expression, we need to work and we need to play, so why should that be any different for a person with dementia? I do not mean we should allow anyone to take real risks, but I believe our fear is blocking a broader vision and a workable solution.

Searching for occupation

Mr A had been observed wandering around a day unit for some time, taking little notice of his surroundings or, indeed, where he was going. Later in the day, he approached the tea trolley and began to wipe out the used cups with his tissue. As soon as staff saw this, he was immediately stopped. From behind, they were unable to see his crestfallen face, the look of dejection, loss of self-esteem.

Five minutes later, Mr A picked up a copy of a book and began to pull at the pages. Thinking he was going to rip the book up, another member of staff tried to take the book away. Mr A struck out at the member of staff. In this case, which was the biggest risk to Mr A and the member of staff?

When I spoke to the staff about the incident, they were unable to explain why he was prevented from wiping the cups. When I suggested that he might be encouraged to help wash up the cups and saucers with a member of staff, I was informed that they were collected by hotel services!

After lengthy discussion, we did manage to turn the situation round – staff became quite positive when I showed them how the incident had disempowered and subsequently affected Mr A. They are now going to incorporate this activity into Mr A's day to facilitate choice and enable his attempts at meaningful occupation to come to fruition.

What's cooking?

During another DCM session within a nursing home, I observed a volunteer leading a 'cookery session' at the table. Wonderful, I thought, residents will be able to participate without any element of risk (they were away from the kitchen, ovens etc). All the residents wore aprons and chefs' hats. All the equipment was laid out on the table – flour, fruit, butter, bowls, cutters, baking trays – and all the residents showed a high level of well-being, chatting to the volunteer and obviously eager to participate. After ten minutes of chatting about things they used to cook and how they did it, the volunteer proceeded to carry out a 'demonstration' – she mixed all the ingredients, cut out all the scones and placed them all on the baking trays, much to the dismay of the residents who intermittently tried to become involved.

As the session progressed, residents' well-being deteriorated and they became totally disengaged – a very different picture from the happy smiling faces I had observed earlier.

Again, I consulted with staff during the feedback and asked why the residents were not involved in the cookery session. Responses varied from 'they might get in a mess', 'the carpet would get in a mess' to 'they may burn themselves'. So I asked, which of these is a real risk and what can we do about it?

Staff concluded that the only actual risk was that people might burn themselves. So why not enable the residents to join in with the weighing, mixing, cutting and placing scones on the tray. Staff would then place them in the oven and retrieve them later.

It seems to me that only when these things are fed back and explained are staff are able to understand the disempowering impact of their actions or inactions. We can find workable solutions to most 'risks' involving creativity and occupation, yet we fail to do so.

We therefore need to broaden our vision. In reality... is it such a risk?

• Published in *JDC*, March/April 2002.

Reference

Bradford Dementia Group (1997) *Evaluating Dementia Care – The DCM Method*. University of Bradford.

16 Is it care... or companionship?

ELIZABETH BARNETT

What does companionship mean? One important fact is that we only consider ourselves to be companions of our fellow human beings. Poets can refer to the companionship of the natural world (such as Wordsworth's daffodils), but in the usual round of everyday living most of us do not normally see ourselves as the companions of trees, houses or the number 10 bus. Trees and buses may (who knows?) be companions to each other, but we who are human tend to consider our companions to be found among the fellow beings of our species. Conversely, therefore, treating a fellow person as if they were an object is automatically to rule them out as candidates for companionship.

In dementia care, those of us familiar with DCM will recall that 'objectification' is one of the 'personal detractions' – the infamous 'PDs' – the 'put downs' which undermine a person's sense of identity and self-worth. To 'objectify' another person is to consign them to the status of non-companions.

The second thing to say about companionship relates to the derivation of the word. Dictionaries refer to companionship in terms of being in fellowship with another, and point to the Latin roots as com or con (with) and panis (bread). This would seem to describe a relationship of shared nourishment.

The listening process

About 10 years ago I began to do research in dementia care. In particular I evaluated a new purpose-built community unit providing support for people with dementia. This consisted of a day hospital, respite and longer term in-patient care, and a base for a community mental health team. I listened to what all the staff, managers and relatives had to say about the unit, but I listened especially to what the elderly clients themselves told me in individual in-depth interviews. And I also used DCM as a way of reading behaviour in an attempt to understand the lived experience of the care provided in the unit. Subsequently, in response to the profound impression which using DCM made on me, I set up a special project which introduced all those involved with the unit to the method. In this way they too were able to share the world of the clients and adapt their practice accordingly.

> **CARE STAFF ARE OFTEN MORE VALUED BY THEIR CLIENTS THAN THEY REALISE, AS IN-DEPTH INTERVIEWING AND MAPPING REVEALED**

'Taking care' and 'looking after' were the phrases most commonly used by staff with regard to their clients. But 'taking care' can easily become 'caretaking,' where a paternalistic (or 'maternalistic') care model leads to a curatorial role for relatives and staff involved. The language we use is not neutral in its effects. It conditions the way we see things and therefore the way in which we behave. For we are curators of objects, but companions of people.

The elderly clients, on the other hand, spoke a great deal of the importance to them of other people. In fact, for over half of them this was the first thing they said. Some examples are quoted in the panel on the next page.

So being surrounded and supported by kind, familiar, friendly people was clearly of great importance to these clients. From my work in this area over the years I have no reason to believe that other elderly clients with dementia place any less significance on fellowship than those I spoke to in Green House. So those of us, as it were, as yet without dementia are greatly valued by those of us, as it were, with dementia. Do those of us (staff, relatives, managers) involved in supporting people with dementia fully appreciate just how much we mean to them?

Transports of delight

Relatives often feel cut off from, and indeed unrecognised by, their loved one with dementia: 'She doesn't know me any more.' And hands-on care staff can often feel themselves unheard and unappreciated by their management. Yet for people with dementia their loved ones and the staff who work in the care environments where they find themselves are clearly enormously important. How sad, therefore, that so often relatives and staff are not aware of just how important they are.

For example, an ironic feature of the Green House research was the fact that the day hospital staff were quite unaware of the extraordinarily high levels of client well-being experienced during the daily journey to and from the day hospital in their minibus, until I began 'mapping.' In fact, all the clients involved demonstrated higher levels of well-being in the minibus than at any other time. So I came to think of these expeditions as 'transports of delight!' From the moment the minibus arrived, each client received a very personalised service. They were greeted by name, with inquiries about themselves, their families, or their homes. They also received quality physical care in helping them get ready for the journey, and onto the minibus.

During the journey they were in a confined space, which naturally intensified the amount of personal interaction; it was not possible for anyone to be left out in such intimate circumstances. Many clients showed evident delight as they greeted and made room for each other. Arrival at the day hospital was the occasion for more physical care as people were helped off the bus, and greeted by the rest of the staff, who came to help them down the little garden path into the entrance. The welcoming cup of tea or coffee rounded off this whole episode with warmth and satisfaction.

Usually the minibus was driven by the hospital porter, with whom everybody had a very friendly relationship. But most interesting of all were the journeys on the porter's day off, when one of the day hospital staff would drive instead. All the staff had been trained to do this, and passed the necessary test. Nevertheless, they were much less familiar with the task.

The small town and surrounding villages served by Green House were characterised by narrow, winding roads, and turning the minibus around in a small lane could become a challenge for all its occupants – staff and clients alike. Clients' eyes and experience were then actually needed, as the travelling microcosm of cared-for and caregivers backed gingerly into gateways and nosed through narrow lanes. The collective sense of achievement after the successful outcome of such adventures was tangible. They all rediscovered in their present experience that, as one of them said, 'we all rely on each other'. Yet the staff had been convinced that journey times were merely a necessary evil, and time subtracted from the really 'therapeutic' activities of the day hospital itself.

Giving and receiving

Once staff began using DCM themselves, they became sensitised to just how valuable their interactions with their clients were. The first change which this led to was an increased focus on mealtimes. These became scenes of much warmth and consideration. Food was the favoured medium of care, because the caring could be seen to be being taken, with enjoyment, into the being of the other. This is, of course, culturally and socially embedded; for instance, our first reaction to a guest tends to be to offer tea and biscuits. But who is being nourished? Is it not mutual? When companions share bread, the giver also receives.

We need, however, to be able to move our companionship of people with dementia beyond the sharing of bread, or,

---

'It's the people that's important'

Interviewer: What about the various things that you do here at Green House? Which of those is particularly enjoyable to you?
Respondent: Well, I think – rather hard to explain – but being among people, talking to them.
[I = Interviewer; R = Respondent]
R: I look forward to coming. And I've met charming people here. Just like coming home again. I like the people. I like the place, but I like the people – attractive people, nice people.
I: It's the people that's important?
R: It is very important anywhere really.
I: That's true.
R: People that make life worth living.

R: I've good friends here.
I: Good friends.
R: Good friends. It's a very good family.
I: Like a family?
R: To feel confidence and to have confidence.
I: So it gives you confidence to feel among friends?
R: Yes!

R: Oh, I like to come here. I like all the people around me because they are known to me.
I: You have got to know them?
R: Oh yes. They are all friendly, very friendly.
I: Sounds as if you look forward to coming.
R: Oh yes. To see all the old faces. Yes. They are all kind. I just like the people. I like everybody here – they are so familiar to me.

---

indeed, other task-oriented situations. The real challenge is learning to 'just be' companionably alongside the person with dementia – without any mediating activity. This means learning to be comfortable in an unstructured situation, often without the reassurance of verbal communication. And we need also to open ourselves to the companionship of those with dementia. Much affection and human concern is already flowing our way; for instance, clients worry about their relatives and about the tiredness of staff. To accept their concern is to honour their fellow humanity. For just as to give is to receive, so to receive is also to give. The love and appreciation which is waiting for us in so many encounters with people with dementia can feed our inner store of feelings of self-worth – and we are then correspondingly enabled to give more back in return. Of course, not all encounters are positive, any more than they are in other field of life; but all the more reason to nurture those that are, or have the capability to be so.

Companionship as a model of care has something positive to offer both those 'with' and those 'without' dementia. Might we one day be reading the Journal of Dementia Companionship?

• Published in *JDC*, March/April 2001.

17 Shining a light on simple, crucial details

TRACY PACKER, VERA BIDDER, JACKIE LEWIS, LAURA MALLER

What were your first thoughts when told about DCM?

L: I had never heard of it before, but when I first went to the introductory training sessions on the ward I thought 'Yeah I can see that!'

V: I was a bag of nerves a few days before, especially as we were only nursing assistants.

J: I didn't understand it at first, and I was really worried because the course was expensive. Having that responsibility was scary. The fact that you had faith in us was good. It was frightening, but we had to trust you: you wouldn't have given us the chance if you didn't think we could do it.

And what was it actually like?

L: The personal introductions were so embarrassing, especially when we stood up in front of everyone to say our names and what we did. I was really aware that we were the only three nursing assistants in attendance alongside clinical psychologists, nursing managers, and occupational therapists.

J: Before we turned up I was really worried about the maths, but when I actually got down to doing it, it was quite simple - it was just so well explained. I helped two other people out in the practice sessions and then I got it wrong in the assessment! I was really annoyed with myself, even though I'd still passed anyway. When the person I helped came and thanked me I felt so chuffed as she was a trained nurse. I had to take my maths GCSE twice so if I could do it, anybody else could.

V: Watching the role play was amazing, Tom Kitwood 'put on' his dementia with his glasses...

J: He just went into the character. There were a couple of times when some of us wanted to get up and help him. There were tears in our eyes and a lump in our throat, but we felt useless because we couldn't actually do anything about it. It was so realistic.

What does it feel like to actually be the person doing the mapping?

J: When I first had a short go at mapping I was very surprised at what I saw. It was a combination of being amazed and confused at the same time. It also seemed quite difficult then.

> **THREE HOSPITAL WARD NURSING ASSISTANTS DESCRIBE THEIR EXPERIENCE OF DEMENTIA CARE MAPPING**

V: It was very frustrating not really being able to intervene and change some things whilst you were the one doing the mapping, although in the back of your mind you knew it would have happened anyway if you weren't actually there.

J: Just through watching what happens on the ward more closely, you know yourself where you need to buck up your own ideas. It really makes you think about all sorts of things. You realise that you are better at some things than others because you also notice plenty of positive feedback, as well as the negative stuff.

V: You wouldn't have always known about the good stuff before, because you would have had so little to go on. Now we can see how things that seem so simple to us, can make such a huge difference to a person with dementia. They can't always speak for themselves and this is one way of helping them get heard. You feel really proud when you see the good results.

How useful was the information you gained from a period of mapping?

L: The 'hands on' practical things were really relevant to us. Although we didn't *have* to do the bar graphs and charts and things, they were helpful, because you could make perfect sense of the information straight away.

V: Shortly after the course I became very conscious of the detractions that were still going on. It still makes me very angry, which is difficult sometimes. I was bathing a person with dementia, who had problems forming a conversation. The door was flung open and the curtain was pulled back. I protested, and the response was 'It's only a patient!' I was livid because I felt like it was me. I was the person having their privacy invaded. I found myself apologising to the person involved even though it wasn't my fault.

J: It's definitely helped me feel stronger. Instead of moaning to another sympathetic colleague all the time and never actually doing anything, I try and diplomatically say something about it myself. I'm very protective about the people I care for now.

V: It will definitely help when a few more staff get to have a go. The more people who learn the better.

J: Yes, they will probably understand why we sometimes seem so fussy. It's as if we have an insight into dementia that we didn't have before, and perhaps we do understand a little more about how it must feel when somebody comes along and treats you like a child.

What did it feel like to be on duty when somebody else was mapping?

J: It felt awful, it felt as if we were being tested all the time.

L: At first it was very difficult to relax when somebody was mapping on the ward, even when you knew you didn't really have anything to worry about...

V: ...but if the 'mappers' had been there for a long time, there would be so many other things that you'd be dealing with, that the last thing on your mind would be what the 'mappers' were watching.

L: You do think that it measures your performance, but it is a good thing because you are so much more conscious of the effect you have on a person with dementia. You apply what you've learned even when you 'disappear' into the toilet with a patient, when no one can actually see or hear what you're doing. It soon starts to become a natural part of what you do every day.

J: There was one time that you had planned to do a mapping and there was 'bedlam' on the ward, but you did it anyway! One member of staff was on an emergency escort, the agency staff hadn't turned up and lots of the morning work had over-run into the afternoon. I was really worried about it.

V: I could have killed you! But when we compared the results with the first one last year – a routine shift with no problems – it was actually better overall, which surprised me. It showed that in spite of all the problems we had on that shift, we had still improved things.

So what changes have you noticed in your own practice now?

L: I've stopped myself from taking over, doing something for a person when they could have done it for themselves. It stemmed from my first job – there were 40 residents who all had to be washed and dressed by nine in the morning, and only six inexperienced nursing assistants. You don't even think about taking time; there's a routine and it must be kept up. Here staff take a lot more time with people.

V: I used to think I was doing something wrong if I took my time, but now I don't have to worry any more.

L: I think I also have more time for a person if I get called over by them.

J: That's true. Before, when I was tending to a patient I used to talk to my colleague about what I was doing last night, or whatever. Now the patient is included in the conversation. Even if they can't answer back in any great detail, at least they're part of it instead of being spoken over.

V: It is so natural, it's not forced now, we do it automatically. It is a routine part of our caring. Also before, I don't think I meant to, but I would only talk to whichever patient I was with at the time. Now I am much more conscious of the people who haven't been obviously involved. Our patients all

used to get sat around the walls, now they sit in small groups. There's conversation and laughter. I'm very careful, I know that if certain people sit together, they will aggravate each other. It makes me think about what I'm doing before I do it.

How have you viewed the ward since the course?

V: After you have done the training I must admit you become very conscious of other members of staff as well as yourself, and you really do notice how things are being said and done. Before, you might have been vaguely aware of it, but you didn't really realise how it might affect the person with dementia. Often that's the way it's always been, somebody who hasn't been on the course won't realise unless we tell them what we've learned; that's our responsibility. The personal detractions and behaviour codings are the most important aspects of the training. We all need to be reminded of those all the time.

L: Let's face it, I didn't know before! The course was like someone shining a little light, and then it seemed so obvious to me. I started off in a place where the care was horrendous. Even when I came here before mapping there was an obvious difference in the way things were done. I've only been an NA for two years, so for me the mapping was another step up.

V: It's improving all the time. We don't seem to get 'aggressive' patients any more. Probably because we understand more about the people we care for, and are able to communicate much more effectively with them. We sometimes get frustrated patients who could potentially become aggressive, but then again that's understandable when you try to imagine what they must be going through. Doing the DCM makes us feel good, we are achieving something that needed to be the open that otherwise would never have been considered.

Is it easy to explain the DCM method to other staff?

V: I had the chance to spend some time with a nursing student who was very interested. She cottoned on to the coding very quickly. Her main concern was with the value judgements and sometimes spotting the personal detractions. It does sometimes seem to be down to your own judgement and I don't think this is something you get over, but the difference is fractional. The more you use the mapping, the more accustomed you get and the easier it is. We noticed on the course that there was a lot of difference at first, between what people thought they saw in the role play, but by the end of it most of us could reach an agreement. At least it actually gets you talking about what you automatically see and do every day, instead of taking things for granted.

J: We could discuss many things that we learned on the course, including the role play which was so real. Talking about the detractions (which I do anyway!) always gets people going.

L: We were very proud to have been the only nursing assistants to have attended and passed.

J: Yes, we all went home with headaches and a smile on our faces!

• Published in *JDC*, Nov/Dec 1996.

18 The effects of DCM on caregiver mappers

ANDREW NEEL

It is over 20 years since I first worked with people with dementia. That was back in the days of the big old psychiatric hospitals, when I was employed as a nursing assistant on night duty. Although I have done other things since then it was that experience which made me want to become a nurse. I continue to find working with people with dementia highly compelling, and I am thrilled by recent developments in dementia care, especially the person-centred approach.

I am very interested in the hidden emotional labour of nursing. By this I mean the way in which we deal with the extreme events that are a commonplace in our work, such as death and bereavement, and also the socially stigmatised things – bodily functions, aggression and violence, madness. In the comments that follow I hope to contribute to the culture of the person-centred approach.

DCM (Kitwood & Bredin 1992; Brooker 2002) is an increasingly widely used method for evaluating dementia care. To give some context to what I have to say about the effects of mapping on caregiver mappers, I will describe the DCM project in the NHS Trust where I work. An initial pilot project in one patient area produced promising results. On the strength of this, a rolling programme was developed for all areas with dementia patients to be mapped and then re-mapped. The long-term aim was to embed the person-centred approach to dementia care in the culture of the trust.

An important characteristic of our project was that, apart from the training which some of us went to Bradford for, everything came from within the Trust. With the exception of one psychologist who was involved in the project, everybody who took part in the actual data gathering was a caregiver, that is either a qualified or auxiliary nurse, whose normal workload consisted of the hands-on delivery of care. We were not experts brought in from outside to carry out a specialist job, but the peers of the caregivers working in the areas we were mapping.

The experience of DCM

What I am interested in here is the experience of those people whose normal day-to-day practice is caregiving when they 'cross the line' and become Dementia Care Mappers. I offer no scientific basis for what follows; it is

THE AUTHOR REFLECTS ON THE HUGE EFFECT DCM HAD ON HIS PERCEPTION OF HIS ROLE AS A NURSE IN DEMENTIA CARE

very largely subjective or based on exchanges with colleagues. I will be merely describing my and our experiences in the hope that they will be recognised and a debate stimulated.

My first experience of DCM was literally shocking. It probably even outstripped my very first experiences in dementia care all those years ago. In many ways, in spite of my attendance on the basic course at Bradford, I felt quite unprepared for this. One had the sense of experiencing something very profound that was too big to be readily assimilated. A full understanding of the meaning and implications of that experience continues to elude me, although on reflection I have made some progress in working out why it should have been quite so shocking.

I now feel sure this was largely due to the extraordinary privilege of being an observer in a setting in which I would normally have an active role. This gave the experience a surreal quality, as if events were taking place at a distance, or through glass, or as if one's own presence had somehow been negated by the radical difference in role – I was there but also not there. It amounted almost to an altered state of consciousness.

Although direct contact with the participant patients is kept to a minimum, I felt a great intimacy with them. It was much more possible to see through the familiar characteristic behaviour of dementia patients to the unique individuals behind the behaviour. I was seeing Kitwood's *people with dementia* rather than 'people with *dementia*'. I realised the extent to which I had accustomed myself to seeing individuals as a series of signs of illness and easily recognisable behaviour patterns. This in itself was a profound disappointment to me – I did not like seeing myself in this light. But it was also quite exhilarating as it felt like the first step in a process of change, a kind of acceptance of the way things are and a realisation of the potential to make them better; an epiphany.

After the initial shockwave described above had died down, there were further areas that were almost as shocking. Although DCM is not overtly concerned with monitoring the performance of caregivers, it was in my observations of them that these secondary shocks were most marked. In the first place I had a strong impression of recognition. In the care practices I observed I saw the clichés of my own practice mirrored, but also stripped bare, without the internal rationalisation that is inherent in so much of what we as caregivers do. I saw my own practice as it is, 'warts and all'. The shock here was akin to the intense embarrassment of seeing oneself on a video recording. Without the stream of internal events – the thoughts and feelings that give meaning to our actions – one is left with the hollow performance, one's behaviour, as others perceive it, good and bad.

Two opposed perspectives

This opened up a contradictory set of emotions, where on one hand I was assessing and judging care according to the rigorous DCM system, and on the other I was rationalising what I saw as an experienced caregiver myself. Inherent in the judgement role was a measure of condemnation.

Care is contingent upon a vast range of extrinsic factors that may not be readily apparent but of which I am aware, at least in general terms. An assumption that underpins DCM is that poor care occurs as a result of ignorance of one sort or another. This is a simplification. I believe poor care is as likely to occur as a result of expediency. Without wishing to labour the point or preach to the converted, dementia care is chronically under-resourced, and has rightly been described as 'the Cinderella of all Cinderella services' (Darby 1999).

What I am describing is a doublethink situation, seeing the same situation from two irreconcilable perspectives simultaneously. Ironically it reminded me of another situation in dementia care. On the one hand the pessimistic, medically dominated 'standard paradigm' (Kitwood 1997), which emphasises the characteristic experience of dementia as loss, is highly valued by many but is worthless in the day to day practice of caring as it actually undermines the value of caring. On the other hand, the more optimistic knowledge base of caregivers is effective but remains poorly valued because much of this knowledge is tacit and difficult to articulate.

Overall, what I am trying to say is that continuing to practice under the competing pressure of two value systems is highly stressful.

A new level of identification

So far I have described shocks related to finding oneself in a familiar environment but in a very unfamiliar role, and to seeing a 'mirror image' of oneself without compensatory defence mechanisms. The third level of shock comes in the unique access to the experience of the participants that DCM provides. The level of identification and empathy with the participants is much greater than I was accustomed to. The most profound sensation here comes not from the individual participants but from the fact that such a disparate group of individuals are gathered together in one place. It is not even that it is a microcosm of society as a whole, but rather it is as if the extremes of society have been shoe-

horned into one space. One is made very aware of the shortcomings in the organisation of dementia care on top of the resource implications.

The overall effect of these successive shocks is very exhausting. One has a sense of having done an extraordinary amount of emotional work. But what one then has to face is the challenge of the next phase of the process – feeding back the results of the evaluation to the staff in the area you have just mapped.

When the results of the evaluation are good, this can be a confirming experience for staff, who often seem to be relieved that a method of assessing their efforts has come into being. They begin to embrace the new concepts and language of DCM and the person-centred approach to care. But when the results are not good, and there are clear inadequacies in the care the participants are receiving, the feedback can become confrontational, staff are angry and defensive, the mappers are identified as arbitrary and cruel. It does not feel as if you are helping. You might hear the sound of cans of worms being opened, and guiltily feel that you are not going to be around to support staff in the long term who are dealing with difficult issues. Staff do not want to accept the information you are giving them. They reject the potential benefits of DCM in general and the feedback process in particular. As a mapper, during feedback, you can feel isolated and vulnerable.

Again it is a doublethink situation. The only reason for your presence is because of your temporary role as Dementia Care Mapper. You are inescapably aware that you would normally be receiving the feedback rather than giving it.

And of course it does not stop there. As well as your activities as a mapper you also still have your practice as a caregiver to contend with, but now with this heightened awareness of self, colleagues and clients. One goes back to familiar ground made strange, with the scales removed from the eyes, with the experience of mapping resonating in the memory. It also has to be said that among your peers in your usual workplace, your involvement in DCM may not be valued. They might interpret your absence from the ward or department as a privilege or soft option, and resent you for it.

Further directions

Tom Kitwood (1997) stressed the need for staff support in general terms, as indeed do other writers (Macdonald 1992, for example), but not specifically in relation to DCM. Tracy Packer (1996) describes interview responses from three nursing assistants about their experience of DCM; this covers some areas that I am interested in. Another article by a group of mappers in Tyne and Wear (Bolton et al 2000) is useful in looking at the support needs of mappers.

As far as our own practice as mappers is concerned, in my trust we are offering support to each other as an inherent part of the process. As for the wider culture of DCM, the first step is to stimulate a debate about this issue, which is what I am trying to do now.

I also believe that training in DCM (at Bradford and elsewhere) should stress the need for support for mappers and try to anticipate some of the emotional difficulties that I have described. Publications like Bradford's manual (Bradford Dementia Group 1997) should reflect this. Possibly this is a reflection of the perspective of the people who developed DCM, who do not come from a background of 'hands-on' care, but have more of a sociological perspective.

Conclusion

My involvement in the DCM programme has been a roller-coaster of highs and lows. So far I have stressed potential problems, all of which have all come from my own experience as a mapper. I offer them in the hope that you will be encouraged to ensure that your own support needs are met during what can be a very trying process.

However, I have also found my involvement in the project to be enormously rewarding and enjoyable. I have met a good number of like-minded people both within the Trust and outside. I have been energised and enthused. My creativity has been encouraged. Most of all, and most personally, I have found a way of becoming the kind of nurse I always wanted to be.

In the past, initiatives to improve care for people with dementia have failed because they have relied on the imagined ability of caregivers to pull themselves up by their own bootstraps. DCM's humanistic ethos means that it avoids this reliance on levitation to a large extent. However, I believe that in the fullness of time the real value of DCM will be as a method of consciousness raising for caregivers to demand the resources they need to do their socially valuable work. I suggest that we grasp this opportunity.

• Published in *JDC*, July/Aug 2002.

References

Bolton J *et al* (2000) Stepping back to move forward with DCM. *Journal of Dementia Care* 8(4) 26-28.

Bradford Dementia Group (1997) *Dementia Care Mapping Manual* (7th edition). University of Bradford, Bradford.

Brooker D (2002) Dementia Care Mapping: a look at its past, present and future. *Journal of Dementia Care* 10 (3) 33-36.

Darby S (1999) Exploring the myths and stereotypes of mental health in old age. In: Darby S, Marr J, Crump A, Scurfield M. *Older people, nursing and mental health*. Butterworth-Heinemann, Oxford.

Kitwood T & Bredin K (1992) A new approach to the evaluation of dementia care. *Journal of Advances in Health and Nursing Care* 1(5) 41-60.

Kitwood T (1997) *Dementia reconsidered: The person comes first*. Open University, Buckingham.

Macdonald A (1992) Home-based case management and the Domus: Models of long-term care of elderly people with dementia and behavioural problems. In: *Department of Health (1992) Long-term care for elderly people: Purchasing, providing and quality*. HMSO, London.

Packer T (1996) Shining a light on simple, crucial details. *Journal of Dementia Care* 4(6) 22-3.

19 DCM training – a carer's perspective

CRESSIDA HAMMATON

I am one of those people who enjoy looking at maps. Someone tells me where they live, or where they are going on their holidays and out comes my atlas. Though I am not all that good at it, I enjoy navigating, and all my life I've carried a compass in my handbag. All this is by way of saying that I like to have a framework, or a set of guidelines to help me on my way when exploring new territory.

> A PERSONAL ACCOUNT OF ENCOUNTERING DCM WITH NO PRIOR THEORETICAL KNOWLEDGE – BUT MUCH PRACTICAL EXPERIENCE

Thus I found myself attending a basic DCM course at Hellesden Hospital in the UK at the beginning of September 2003. My route there had been via my interest in dementia as my husband had been slowly losing some of his mental faculties over some years, finally ending up in a nursing home for the last seven months of his life.

I am not young myself and I left school without going to college, so I am unfamiliar with any form of further education, let alone studying a course. I went because I had read some of Tom Kitwood's work and I knew instinctively that I'd found someone whose approach to dementia was not only innovative but inspired. His work in this area had not seeped through the system to be of help to my husband. My husband was one of many, but the many matter as much as the one.

It was therefore with some trepidation that I set out for Hellesden. Would my mind work for me under discipline? Would I be able to keep up with others and stay the course? Despite being the eldest and not in employment I was made to feel welcome.

A person with dementia is not a demented person – I discovered that while living with my husband Peter. Tom Kitwood's approach of person-centred care was amply illustrated on my first day of the course. I felt at home. Mapping, I discovered, is a science based on minute observation. It's a way of charting one's voyage through a sea of unknown. How do we know what someone needs if that someone does not have a way of expressing him or herself as we do? I sometimes felt as if I were in another dimension with Peter. The rulebook had gone out of the window; I could only feel my way and have no expectations, as life was full of the unexpected. I began to realise that mapping is a way of pin-pointing one's exact location, it's immediate and allows one to see, by the behaviour of the persons involved, both what is lacking and what is positive in their interaction. The course leaders Judith and Paul illustrated this fact with well-thought-through scenarios and I re-lived the many times I had visited Peter. They brought tears to my eyes.

I had expected the course to be a blackboard-and-taking-notes situation, which would not have done me much good as I always find it hard to decipher my scribblings. Instead we were all fully participating every step of the way – rather like hands-on science, which is becoming more popular these days. What really helped me was the handbook: it had everything I needed to know in it. So homework was simply a matter of re-reading the handbook and gathering up bits I had missed. Mapping at first felt like a bit of a maze, but unlike a maze, this one had signposts; all I needed to do was learn how to use them. There was also a certain amount of calculation to be done, a kind of summing up of experiences into visible form. I was slow at that. It occurred to me that if I wanted to practice on that aspect I could map some of the family. I'm sure it could throw light on family interactions.

I felt at the end like a pioneer – a good feeling that engages my heart as well as my brain. Like all breakthroughs, time is needed for the 'good news' to filter down through the system. The home where Peter lived was understaffed at times, they have a mountain of physical work to do which leaves little time for establishing relationships, they are short of money and many of their 'inmates' have been abandoned by their families. I understand this; it's easy to be totally out of one's depth caring for people who seem to have lost their way. Help is needed all round.

I think sometimes that despite the loss of Peter and the grief that goes with that, he has left a small nugget of pure gold, a hope that others like him will one day be able to live out their lives with dignity and full personhood.

20 Improving DCM feedback sessions

LORNA MACKENZIE, IAN JAMES, LESLIE LEE

This report outlines a set of guidelines designed to improve the quality of the feedback provided to staff working in residential homes following a DCM session. The guidelines were developed from information obtained from two separate studies.

> WITHOUT REFLECTIVE FEEDBACK TO STAFF THERE IS LITTLE POINT IN DOING DCM

The first study involved an empirical investigation on effective staff feedback. The other study examined video-tapes of staff engaged in role-playing DCM feedback sessions. The guidelines were initially developed for a workshop (James 2001) run to enhance people's confidence and competence with respect to this potentially difficult aspect of the DCM process.

Gathering feedback

As part of the mapping procedure, a feedback session is organised by the mappers undertaking the DCM procedure, at which point the results of the monitoring are presented. The aim of the feedback session is to acknowledge and reinforce evidence of good practice, and to identify and provide constructive help in areas found wanting. Owing to the obvious sensitivities involved, the sessions often pose difficulties for those giving, and those receiving, the feedback. The following protocol was developed to facilitate this process.

The feedback process is in many respects the most important feature of the DCM procedure. Indeed, it is through appropriate feedback that staff are able to reflect on examples of good practice, practices that need to be changed and how change can take place. However, from personal experience, and discussions with people who attended the Bradford DCM course (the national training course in DCM), it was felt that we were not prepared sufficiently to conduct feedback sessions, based on the training provided during the course.

It is relevant to note that the Bradford course has clearly outlined the importance of this aspect of DCM. Indeed, based on personal correspondence, we are aware that Bradford Dementia Group is currently making efforts to improve the teaching of feedback on the Basic DCM Course.

The present guidelines, shown in Tables 1 and 2 on the following pages, are an extension of a clinical psychology doctorate project conducted by Stepney (2000) and a product of a workshop run at the Centre for Health of the Elderly, Newcastle General Hospital.

The workshop

The workshop was organised by a clinical psychologist (IJ) and a G grade RMN (LL). Both had attended the Bradford DCM course. LL was a very experienced, advanced DCM mapper.

It was attended by eight people from Newcastle City Health Trust, who were graduates of the Bradford DCM course. They were all experienced mappers, but none had provided feedback to staff. This situation had arisen because they had previously been using DCM as an outcome measure within a research study, and not as an instrument for implementing changes to working practices.

As part of the needs assessment of the workshop, roleplay scenarios were conducted by the second author (IJ) to determine the features that needed to be focused on during the teaching. As part of the role play, the participants were given data concerning an imaginary mapping session (well-/ill-being (WIB) scores; personal detractions; positive events, etc). The participants were then asked to give feedback using this data, with IJ taking on the role of a member of staff receiving the feedback. All of the role plays were videotaped. They were examined in terms of style and content, and the information gleaned proved useful in designing the teaching programme and producing the guidelines.

In general the feedback was of a good standard, but some key principles of communication and learning were not being followed during the roleplay sessions:

• Too much information was being given during the session. This was causing difficulties for both the person giving the feedback and the recipient. For example, the mapper was often rushing through the material, and the recipient was not being given time to assimilate it

• There was insufficient summarising with respect to the key points, which prevented opportunities for appropriate reflection and discussion

• There was insufficient reinforcement of good examples of behaviour

• A lot of DCM jargon was used (eg WIB values, personal detractions, etc) *(continued on page 64)*

Guidelines for a DCM Feedback Session

General features

Preparation

Remember the goal of the DCM is to improve well-being values by identifying and targeting staff/resident interaction. Thus, whatever type of information is fed back (numbers, means, detractions, etc), it must be aimed at improving staff interaction. So do not cloud issues by giving irrelevant material.

- Avoid jargon
- Reflect on the content of the feedback and think about how different members of the staff team (qualified nurses, nursing assistants, etc) may be feeling about receiving it
- Review the results of the mapping and decide what can be realistically changed at that point in time, in that setting, with that group of staff. For example, choose two detractions that can be targeted. By having specific and well-defined targets for change, you are better able both to focus on managing change within the whole unit and to ensure that the change is lasting
- Decide what words you are going to use for feeding back negative information (poor interactions, unhelpful actions, etc). The choice of words should be clear and unambiguous, but also sensitive and diplomatic.

Style

- Set up a good alliance with the staff (good verbal and non-verbal communication skills)
- Pace the session appropriately
- Reinforce the positive staff interactions
- Distance and depersonalise the negative aspects
- Provide regular and specific summaries of what has been said
- Be collaborative and non-prescriptive, allowing the staff to reflect on their own behaviour. Ask them about the anxieties of being mapped, and how this may have influenced the behaviour observed
- Allow the staff to discuss the obstacles that they encounter when trying to deliver a good service (eg If we only had more information about Bob; If the room was larger; If I could sit with him: If there were more people on the shift, etc). Such reflection can result in staff suggesting alternative approaches that could be used to facilitate discussion of detractions
- Allow staff to discuss the challenges they can face with specific residents. For example, by allowing them to discuss the problems with coping with 'Bob', they may be more receptive during the discussion about the detractions witnessed with him. Having been allowed to ventilate their difficulties, the staff are often more willing to engage in an open debate about better ways of interacting with him.

Structural features

Introduction

- Thank the staff for their time
- Acknowledge the difficulties of being observed
- Outline the goals of the feedback session. Inform the group that you will feed back information about the following issues:
- Meaningful activities (A-Z of day-to-day activities) of resident
- Positive interactions
- Unhelpful interactions
- Ask the staff what they want to get from the session (ie a needs assessment), checking also whether the staff have any questions regarding the goals of the session.

Results

- It is often helpful to present the information in a visual form, eg. as a graph (see Figure 1 and associated text overleaf)
- Discuss the range of meaningful activities
- Discussion of positive interactions
1. Start with an example of a positive interaction and end with a positive example
2. Use graphs, outlining sequences of interaction that highlight the message you want to give. For example, if you are targeting 'disempowerment', present a period of time where there are examples of both 'disempowerment' and 'empowerment'
3. Praise the positive aspects of an interaction
4. Personalise the praise. For example, 'Joan provided an excellent example of empowerment here. She did X, Y and Z.' Try to say something positive about everyone in the group, if at all possible. One needs to be careful not to cause resentment through this process. Hence, it is often useful to examine the qualities in the rest of the team that may have given Joan the opportunity (time, etc) to experience these positive things
5. Highlight the important skills being displayed by the staff
6. Ask the staff to put themselves in the place of the person with dementia, and to reflect on how this person would have felt during the positive and negative interactions.

- Discussion of negative interactions
1. Examine the unhelpful aspects
2. Depersonalise these issues – avoid picking individuals out for criticism. Use general statements.
3. Examine the issues in terms of what needs to be changed
4. It is often useful to compare the notions of realistic versus ideal. For example: 'If you had all the resources, and all the time, what would you do in this situation?', 'Now based on what resources you do have, how close can you get to what you'd ideally want to do?'
5. Plan exactly how to execute changes
6. Summarise decisions.

- Discussion of 'challenging' residents
1. Often, when you go into a home there is one or more person with dementia that the staff generally find difficult to manage. Sometimes the mapper can get drawn into focusing excessively on this person. However, attempt to avoid focusing on one individual too much, as he/she may not be representative of the other residents
2. If you must focus on the issue of a particular person, ask the staff to identify which member of staff gets on with him/her the best. Then ask the reasons for the better level of interaction between the two individuals. Use this member of staff's behaviour as a template for the others.

Ending

- Present a clear summary of the positive outcomes
- Clarify the things that need to be changed, plan how the change can be carried out and monitored
- Agree a realistic time frame during which progress towards goals can be reviewed.

Example dialogue used with graph in feedback session

Here is an example of how to use the graph. Owing to time considerations, you might choose to do this with only one or two residents. This text provides some dialogue regarding a resident called Bob. He was reported by staff as being one of the most 'problematic'. He would often sit for long periods with his head in his hands. Sometimes he would sit by himself and gently sob. (Italics = staff speech.)

• I'd just like to give an overview of the bit of the mapping that I am going to be concentrating on today. This re-run of the events will help to remind you of what happened two weeks ago when we did the mapping.

As you can see, Bob seemed to be really enjoying watching the game of cards. However, his mood really dropped here, when people were being taken for dinner and he was by himself. When Joan sat and spoke to him, he seemed much brighter. But when someone came over to ask him to choose items from the menu, he became anxious again. He remained upset for the next 20 minutes. From my notes, I see that he was sitting at the corner of the table by himself. Then Lucy came across and had a brief chat, and helped him move into the lounge.

Now I'd like to concentrate on those things that made Bob's mood change. Obviously, the longer he stays in the top half of the graph 'the better' for him. So let's look at what things kept his mood up at the top, and what things made him move down into the bottom section.

As you all know Bob well, can you tell why he was so happy at point 1?

• *He likes being with people. Bob can have great fun, without actually doing anything – just watching things.*

• So he likes being around people. Yeah, it was interesting that he wasn't directly involved in the game, but he was enjoying it. So what do you think he was getting from doing that?

• *I think it's the contact with people. Someone smiles at him and he smiles back. In truth, I don't think he understands what's going on, or always what's being said. He likes being on the periphery. I think he'd find it difficult if he was at the centre of things.*

• So he seems to be a very sociable man, but would rather not be the centre of attention. It is interesting to note that this view seems to be borne out by what was happening at point 6. But we'll come to that later.

• Here (point 2), he is now sitting by himself and his mood has plummeted. From the other profiles I can see that at this time other people were being taken in for lunch. He seems to have been left by himself in the lounge. Is that a regular thing or something that happened on that day?

• *Well, because of his wheelchair, it's easier to move him last of all. But it is true that he often gets distressed when he's by himself. It's as if he doesn't know what's happening. I think he gets a bit confused.*

• Yeah, I agree, I don't think he knew what was happening. Lots of people were walking past him, and he was trying to catch someone's eye – perhaps for reassurance. I wrote down that he was being ignored.

Is there any way we could help Bob if a similar situation arose again.

• *I suppose we could move him in first. He'd be by himself at the table for a short while – but not for long.*

• That sounds a good idea. But say there was some reason he needed to be left by himself. Is there anything we could do differently next time in order to reduce his confusion?

• *I suppose that we could tell him that it was his turn next, and that we weren't leaving him behind.*

• That sounds really good. Now, at point 3 his mood shoots up. Joan comes over, kneels down to him and says something. His mood really improves. Can you remember what you said Joan?

• *No, not really. It was two weeks ago!*

• But what do think you might normally say to him in this sort of situation to brighten him up. Because I see from the notes that when you chat to him, his mood often goes up. There's obviously something that you are doing that is really effective. Knowing what you're doing may help the rest of us deal with Bob better. Let's talk a little more about this...

This excerpt demonstrates the sort of style that might be used. Clearly it is time consuming, but because it is a far more thorough and detailed approach, it has a greater capacity to initiate and maintain appropriate change. It uses a collaborative style with respect to staff engagement, encouraging the staff to become involved in a problem-solving way of thinking.

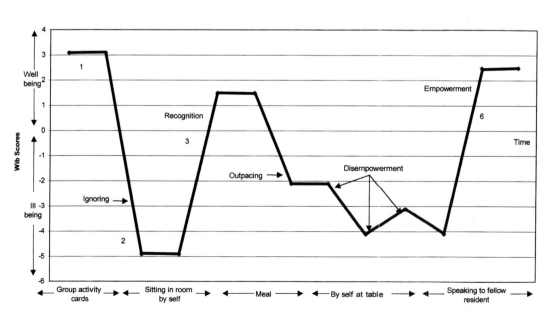

Figure 1: Typical graph for an individual during a DCM session

• There was too much focus on numbers, scores and mean values. It was evident that when faced with so many numbers and mapping jargon that the staff would find the material too difficult to comprehend fully.

The information obtained from the videotape material, along with the key principles obtained by Stepney (2000), were used in the development of the guidelines set out opposite. The guidelines are presented in terms of both general and structural features with respect to the nature of the presentation.

Conclusion

A mapping procedure is both an audit process and a method for improving the care of people with dementia. As Kitwood (1997) has articulated, the well-being of the person with dementia is greatly dependent on the qualities of the interactions the person has with his/her context and environment. The nature of the interactions that people have with others is paramount in this respect, due to the fact that humans are social beings. Hence, it is essential that we promote good relationships between staff and residents in order to enhance the personhood of both. As outlined above, the feedback procedure is the main feature of DCM designed to initiate change. Hence, it is important that we deliver it as effectively as possible. The aim of this paper has been to raise the issue and make some practical suggestions regarding its delivery.

• Published in *JDC*, Sept/Oct 2002.

References

James IA (2001) *Workshop on DCM feedback*. Centre for the Health of the Elderly. Newcastle General Hospital, Newcastle-upon-Tyne: August (unpublished guidelines).

Kitwood T (1997) *Dementia Reconsidered. The person comes first*. Open University Press, Buckingham.

Bradford Dementia Group (1997) *Evaluating Dementia Care: The DCM Method*, 7th ed. Bradford Dementia Group, University of Bradford.

Stepney J (2000) *The use of Dementia Care Mapping as a supervision tool*. Doctoral thesis, Department of Clinical Psychology. University of Newcastle, UK.

Acknowledgements

Thank you to Dawn Brooker for her helpful comments regarding an early draft of the paper. Also, thanks to Margaret Ayton, Senior Commission Manager for NMET Local Levy Fund, for helping to finance the workshop on which this work was based.

21 The role of the 'trusted stranger' in DCM feedback

CHRISTIAN MÜLLER-HERGL

Nearly 1,000 people have been trained in DCM in Germany since its introduction there in 1998 As usual, interest seems to surpass application. But within Germany we are gaining considerable insights into the disadvantages and advantages of the method and its effects within care organisations.

DCM as an instrument and a method is a vehicle for the development of person-centred care. Drawing on social rather than medical models of dementia, DCM shapes awareness of what people with dementia supposedly do and feel. Feedback given by a 'trusted stranger' (see box overleaf) to staff is supposed to trigger a learning process among the team.

This article outlines some of the challenges about the feedback process. Feedback rests on the assumption that trusted strangers can distance themselves from the work. Feedback relies on organisational and management support to develop the role of the mapper and to enable team development. In reality, feedback often leads to 'enlightened misery' without support to develop skills across the team and care organisation.

It is difficult to tell care staff about what a dementia care mapper has observed. In my view DCM is only of use to mature institutions which have already addressed the issues involved in delivering person-centred care. The question then is whether DCM is what such well-developed institutions need? For institutions at the beginning of their development DCM may be of no great use or help.

It is easy to forget how difficult it is to fully understand the behaviour of an individual with dementia. Although we are taught that personality, biography, neurological impairment and health all play essential roles in determining how each individual is affected by dementia, we assume in DCM that apathy, withdrawal and challenging behaviour are due primarily to social neglect. This means we may lose track of the impact of such actions and behaviours and the fact that they have many interpretations.

Signs of illness and coping strategies are the result of one's way of life but also symptoms of disease. For example, if we label social withdrawal as a problem, we are treating a value judgement as if it is a fact. The person is presented as withdrawn, with the implication that

> USING DCM IN CARE SETTINGS BRINGS MANY CHALLENGES, ESPECIALLY IN THE FEEDBACK PROCESS

something has to be done. However, there may be many explanations for this state. Maybe the person has always led a withdrawn, socially isolated life? Maybe silence is their way of controlling the situation, of retreating to an inner self? Maybe it is the intolerable present? Maybe the immediate effects of psychological changes in the brain, or an unknown but unspeakable grief best left alone? Maybe the person only appears to be withdrawn but is in fact keenly listening? This deserves respect and only possibly intervention.

A better way to present this is not in the form of the well-being of another person (ascribing feelings to them) but in the form of a description of our own feelings as a mapper: 'she strikes me as if she could be in need of...' or 'my own feelings observing her struck me as...'. This is what most experienced mappers do. But on paper you have identified a problem and this means we forget it has been interpreted subjectively. We may be mistaken. We may have projected our own feelings on to the person observed.

Understanding versus control

Observation and feedback follow a different logic from that of caring processes within institutions. They require an understanding approach which is only of limited relevance when care tasks have to be done. Within institutions, the day-to-day work rules the day. For neither staff nor residents is it possible to differentiate between their own wishes and the institution's demands. The nurse does not want to make residents go to bed in the early evening but thinks, maybe wrongly, that she has to do this. Likewise, residents learn that the nurse will be happy if they go to bed early, and even seem to want it.

Some staff strive towards person-centred care within the 'care machine' by creating little islands that nourish professional ideals. They create special occasions to 'go the extra mile', move to the night shift, or try to change their practice with individuals. It is generally left to the individual member of staff whether and how to personalise relationships.

Small worlds develop their own subcultures and tend to see everything from the outside as 'alien' (doctors, relatives, inspectors, researchers, mappers). The splitting

The trusted stranger

The role model for a mapper must be an outsider but not an 'expert'. This person must challenge but understand, be experienced in dementia care on a daily basis but rooted in the belief that changes are always possible. Such a person gives little attention to visions and ideologies but develops together with the team the very next step with regard to their daily practice, the setting and further training.

of 'inner and outer' reflects the position of the home as a negative container. Outsiders (these could be people doing DCM) disturb established routines, rituals and power.

Keeping the machine going needs a plan that organises the day into an effective purposeful system. Nursing plans, meal plans, plans for seating, for activities, for outings, for baths, for breaks, for rest – you name it! A person's wishes might become part of a plan. But anyone who seems to go against the plan can be seen as very difficult by staff. The system expects that residents will be humble participants, that they will not make too many demands and will resign themselves to their fate. The plan, not the individual, is central to the organisation.

Staff working in institutional settings create order. Focusing on physical care is a way of coping with an over-complex situation. Getting things straight is also a way for staff to orientate themselves, not necessarily the person with dementia. Staff strive towards order because order is constantly at the brink of collapse. This results in limited contact with people with dementia ('I'll be back in a minute', 'I don't know right now', 'maybe tomorrow') or avoidance behaviour (for example, by rushing past them, or going off to have a smoke). This is illustrated by the common behaviour of us all, perhaps: talking but at the same time reaching for the door handle.

Being caught up in an emotionally charged climate, staff swing between action (to create order) and refusal. Observation from outside, awareness and attention to the shadow side of care, accepting what we do not understand, identifying with individuals, reflecting on what is done – all these remain a strange intrusion into the world of work. Many, if not most, staff enmeshed in institutions find it difficult to identify with a procedure such as DCM that opens up the small world to public view or makes us think about what we are doing.

All this does not mean that DCM feedback is impossible, but shows some reasons why the number of institutions using it regularly over long periods of time is still quite small. In most institutions, the resistance against feedback and the learning that goes with it are stronger than the will and power of change agents.

Roles

Two questions arise. What position does a mapper need to adopt to provide effective feedback? Under what conditions is it possible that a team will benefit from DCM? If the mapper is an 'insider', there will be anxiety about upsetting colleagues. Avoidance of conflict results in uninteresting feedback. DCM is carried out for the sake of it and nobody seems to learn anything.

If the mapper is an 'outsider', they will know little about residents, the team and institution. Professional outsiders or 'experts' are expensive, do not come on a regular basis and are either cheered as redeemers (who will necessarily disappoint) or another of those experts who never fully understand the lack of resources, of training, or ability, of the tiredness, the strain and so on. External experts may be necessary at the start but often leave teams in 'enlightened misery'. The team now knows how bad it is but does not have the means or courage to change it.

The role model for a mapper must accordingly be an outsider but not an 'expert'. This person must challenge but understand, be experienced in dementia care on a daily basis but rooted in the belief that changes are always possible. Such a person gives little attention to visions and ideologies but develops together with the team the very next step to take with regard to their daily practice, the setting and further training. We are trying to address this framework for reflective practice within Germany.

Regional learning in Germany

The German Ministry of Health has supported a DCM regional learning network from January 2002 in the following four regions (figures are approximate):
- Aachen – population 240,000; 14 institutions
- Brandenburg – population 75,000; 6 institutions
- Main-Kinzig-Kreis – population 400,000; 10 institutions
- Marburg-Biedenkopf – population 250,000; 15 institutions.

The model projects are running for 3 years. In each region 10-15 nursing homes have agreed to cooperate in a project of DCM-supported learning. The homes are connected in sets of two or three (A sends mappers to B, B to C, C to A). Grouping homes together in this way means mappers do not have to map in their own facility but can establish themselves as 'trusted strangers' for others. The groupings change every year.

Mappers are qualified nurses who receive further training in dementia care to develop this role. In the participating homes, all staff receive elementary training in dementia care. Trainers teach and train while working with the teams providing care. In the first year supervisors accompany mappers and teams to develop a culture of giving and listening feedback and to set up and implement action plans. The regional government provides resources for this process; there are regular meetings of the mappers, regular meetings of all home managers, regional meetings between regional government representatives and the supervisors of teams and mappers. Each year a guide to best practice will be published for other institutions to learn from.

Within this structure we hope some of the mappers will

develop the role of 'trusted stranger' for other institutions and become reflective practitioners in their own. The structure of the model clarifies rights and responsibilities for each participant in the form of a contract of commitment. This provides different levels of support and consultation. Up to now the most helpful element of the model seems to be the presence of supervisors. This highlights my earlier point that DCM requires a mature style of communication and interaction. The second most helpful element

seems to be interest from the regional government's coordinator. This position provides not only networking but also public relations, and the project has had an impact on the priorities of home inspectors and funders.

The project group that launches this model hopes that we can work towards a change in the culture of caring that addresses not only people, but structure, regulations and funding. Within this framework DCM makes a lot of sense.

• Published in *JDC*, March/April 2004.

22 Using DCM and Engagement to audit care quality

DAWN BROOKER

Dementia Care Mapping (DCM) (Kitwood & Bredin 1992; Bradford Dementia Group 1997) has now emerged as the audit tool of choice in assessing the quality of care for people with dementia in formal care settings (Brooker et al 1998). Before this, many service evaluators used levels of service user engagement in some form or other, to good effect. Unlike Dementia Care Mapping, the evaluation of engagement was not underpinned by a significant theory other than 'being active is better than being inactive'. Before the advent of DCM, however, this was one of the few ways in which the experience of people with dementia could be fed into service evaluations or the quality assurance process. Much of this work was unpublished, partly because the work was small scale and partly because the trend in published research in dementia care has only recently changed to consider papers with a less directly medical perspective.

I have had the experience of running two large scale quality assurance cycles, one using Engagement and one using DCM as its main measure of quality of life. I have concluded that, while DCM is more costly in terms of initial investment, the resultant quality of data far outstrips that of engagement data when improving the quality of care for individuals is the main consideration. Engagement has the advantage, however, that it is usually possible to include all residents in a unit (in DCM the focus is on just a few). It is also relatively easy to learn how to do reliably compared to DCM. Engagement levels may suffice if all that is required is an overall indicator of service quality. Borrowing an image from the world of maps, it can be useful to think of DCM as an Ordnance Survey Map (a lot of detail in a little area) and engagement measures as a Road Map of the UK (much less detail but a larger spread).

There is some data to suggest that there is a correlation between WIB scores as measured in DCM and level of engagement (Brooker et al 1998). This is also reported in this article. I do think there is scope for combining the two methodologies – which will provide a richer picture of the lives of people within formal dementia care settings. This article sets out to say why this may be advantageous, and suggests a way of doing thus. First I will describe the engagement method and its usefulness in describing service quality.

> COMBINING DCM AND ENGAGEMENT CAN PROVIDE A ADDITIONAL INDICATOR OF QUALITY OF LIFE

Engagement methodology

Structuring observations in terms of engaged or disengaged behaviours has been practised for many years (McClannahan & Risley 1975; Jenkins et al 1977; Felce et al 1980; McCormack & Whitehead 1981; Godlove et al 1982; McFayden 1984) The method is based on the simple assumption that if a person is engaged (interacting) with their environment they are likely to be leading a more satisfying life than a person who is disengaged for long periods of time. Bond & Bond (1990) observed that in environments where care is less institutionalised, engagement in activity is higher.

Early engagement evaluations simply consisted of a percentage head count of service users engaged in activity and those who were disengaged, using a momentary time sampling observation technique. This method of measuring engagement described by Felce et al (1980) was extended by McFayden (1984) who further delineated the categories of engaged or disengaged behaviour. McFayden demonstrated that, with minimal training (20-30 observations), satisfactory levels of inter-rater reliability could be achieved. He also showed that the measure was stable over time (six months apart).

Engagement as a quality indicator

Studies which have measured engagement (McFayden 1984; Bond & Bond 1990) report very low levels of activity (typically 20-30 per cent) in elderly care environments. A more recent comparison of two units using engagement type observations confirm that this depressing picture has not changed (Nolan et al 1995).

In the published literature, significant increases in engagement have only been demonstrated as a direct result of activities being provided (McClannahan & Risley 1975; Jenkins et al 1977; McCormack & Whitehead 1981). All the published work to date has only measured engagement at one or two points in time.

I managed an NHS Quality Assurance Cycle during which 250 McFayden type engagement profiles were completed over eleven evaluations in continuing care, assessment wards and day hospital settings (Brooker 1994). Momentary time sampling observations were made every ten minutes of all service users in public areas on the various units. Observations were made manually and recorded on a raw data sheet. Observations were made from 9am to 6.30pm in all the studies and extended to 10pm where possible. In order to ensure that the observations were reliable all observers were personally trained by me. A one-hour period of observation was assessed to ensure inter-rater reliability at each evaluation.

The percentage of time that each individual spent in different behavioural categories over the day was calculated. Thus, each service user had ten 'scores' representing each behavioural category. The average group percentage of time engaged in the different behavioural categories was also calculated. Changes in these percentages over time for each facility were taken to be a rough index of service quality.

It is not the purpose of this paper to provide an exhaustive breakdown of levels of engagement over the various cycles. Taken as a whole, however, some interesting patterns did emerge.

The first time engagement measures were recorded on the assessment ward they were found to be very similar to other published reports, eg an average of 20-30% across the day. A number of quality improvements were made, including increased staffing levels and improved skill mix (including increased occupational therapy and psychology staff), regular staff training and induction, the establishment of various activities for patients, and clearer management and consultation for all staff.

After this first year a culture of continuous quality improvements was aimed at, using the staff and service user feedback interviews (Brooker & Dinshaw 1998). In subsequent evaluations engagement levels of 50-60% were regularly achieved within assessment ward and day hospital settings, and 30-40% was achieved on continuing care and respite care units.

These sorts of levels were adopted as bench marks of quality within the different settings. The averages rarely rose above the top figures of 60% in assessment/day hospitals and 40% in continuing care/respite care. However, a significant decrease on these figures was always carefully scrutinised and reasons sought to explain it. Decreases were usually seen as the result of increases in dependency levels, staff changes, staff shortages or changes in unit activity programmes.

Although the level of engaged behaviour varied over the different evaluations, the pattern remained very similar, with the highest levels recorded at meal times and the lowest levels generally before or after meals. Generally levels of engagement fell slightly during the evening.

The relationship between Engagement and DCM

A comparison between the Behaviour Categories within McFayden Engagement Categories and the Behaviour Category Coding within DCM is problematic. Many of the Engagement Categories (of which there are 10) include multiple DCM categories (of which there are 24). A more straightforward comparison can be made between WIB scores and percentage of time engaged in any activity. Brooker et al (1998) found a strong positive correlation between the percentage of time people were engaged and individual WIB (well-being/ill-being) scores. It should be emphasised that this finding is based on a small amount of data (ten individuals). It may be that over a longer period the correlation would weaken or strengthen. This will only be shown by further empirical study in this area.

A positive correlation is not surprising as there is much within the DCM method that emphasises activity and interaction. If we extrapolate from this data it suggests that an engagement level of around 40% equates to an individual WIB score of+1.0, 60% equates to +2.0 and 80% to a +3.

Combining Engagement and DCM

There are two developments which I feel are worth pursuing in combining DCM and Engagement measures. The first area is where time is limited but decisions need to be made about quality of care. Two typical examples of this would be in inspection of services, and in research. The second area is in enriching the data when undertaking a routine DCM evaluation.

a) Inspection and research

The correlation between engagement levels and Individual WIB Scores lends weight to the assertion that there is a link between engagement in activity and well-being. Engagement Levels could be a simpler and quicker method for indicating the general quality of services for simple research or inspection purposes.

Inspection teams are often at a loss as to how to evaluate the experience of care for people with dementia, and they are not in a position to carry out DCM. Observing engagement levels at key times such as over a main meal and the period directly afterwards could provide teams with useful information on the well-being of people with dementia in formal care settings. This could be strengthened still further by combining the observations with formal recording of any Personal Detractors and Positive Events. For example, if they were observing levels of engagement of under 20% combined with high levels of Personal Detractors and low levels of Positive Events, the inspectors might want to suggest that the care setting considers doing DCM or thinking about how they could improve the quality of care. This is an area for further field work and research.

b) Enriching Dementia Care Maps

A criticism that is often levelled at DCM is that it only captures the experience of a limited number of service users. This is particularly true where there is only one person available to map, as data for only five individuals can be collected reliably. By having detailed maps of five

Date: 20.10.97 Time Period: 9.30–11.30 Place: Courtmeadow No. of Participants: 19 No. of staff: 3 Observer: DB

Participant Name		9.30	9.35	9.40	9.45	9.50	9.55	10.00	10.05	10.10	10.15	10.20	10.25	10.30	10.35	10.40	10.45	10.50	10.55	11.00	11.05	11.10	11.15	11.20	11.25	ΣWIB	ΣTF
Reg C	BCC	P	F	F	L	B	F	F	N	F	F	A	P	M	N	B	B	E	E	K	K	F	F	F	M	42	24
	WIB	+1	+3	+3	+1	+1	+3	+3	+1	+1	+1	+1	+3	+1	+1	+1	+1	+1	+1	+1	+3	+3	+3	+1	+3		
Frank S	BCC	B	M	M	A	F	A	F	O	F	F	M	M	B	M	M	M	M	M	O	A	F	K	K	B	34	24
	WIB	+1	+3	+1	+3	+3	+1	+1	+1	+1	+1	+1	+1	+1	+1	+1	+1	+1	+1	+1	+1	+1	+1	+1	+1		
George D	BCC	W	W	B	B	B	F	W	A	F	F	B	B	W	W	A	W	W	A	W	W	W	W	W	W	34	24
	WIB	+1	+1	+1	+1	+1	+3	+1	+1	+3	+1	+1	+1	+1	+1	+3	+1	+1	+3	+1	+1	+1	+1	+1	+1		
Joe	BCC	M	F	F	B	A	F	B	A	F	F	B	A	A	K	K	K	E	E	F	C	A	A	A	A	56	24
	WIB	+1	+3	+1	+1	+1	+1	+1	+3	+1	+1	+1	+3	+3	+3	+1	+3	+5	+5	+5	-1	+3	+1	+3	+3		
Hazel	BCC	A	A	F	F	F	F	F	F	B	B	A	P	K	K	W	O	W	C	C	C	A	F	F	B	44	24
	WIB	+1	+1	+5	+5	+1	+3	+5	+3	+1	+1	-3	-1	+1	+3	+1	+1	+1	-1	+3	-1	+3	+1	+1	+1		

11.00 Joe's wife visits

Engagement Data

	9.30	9.35	9.40	9.45	9.50	9.55	10.00	10.05	10.10	10.15	10.20	10.25	10.30	10.35	10.40	10.45	10.50	10.55	11.00	11.05	11.10	11.15	11.20	11.25	Percentage of 'engaged' observations
Number of non-DCM participants engaged	3	3	5	4	6	8	8	6	7	6	6	6	6	6	4	5	7	7	7	4	4	3	2	2	
Number of non-DCM participants disengaged	7	7	7	8	7	4	2	7	7	8	8	8	8	7	9	8	7	6	5	9	10	11	12	12	$\frac{126}{309} = 41\%$
Number of non-DCM participants in time frame	10	10	12	12	13	12	10	13	14	14	13	13	13	14	13	12	13	10	11	12	14	14	14	14	Total of non-DCM observations 309

70

individuals and recording levels of engagement of the other residents on a unit would add to the richness of the data that could be presented back to the staff team.

Experience on an Advanced DCM course suggests that it is possible to combine the two methods using the modified data sheet shown on the previous page. Engagement, in this context, is defined simply as interaction occurring between the individual and their external environment. This includes any obvious activity (Type I categories) and Walking (K) and Watching (B). Disengagement is where there is no obvious interaction (CDNUWY) with the outside world or where there is clear evidence of distress. Engagement calculations are based on time sampling 'snap-shot' observations. Imagine you were taking a photograph of the person at regular intervals. On seeing that snap-shot the mapper decides whether individuals were interacting with their environment (engaged) or not (disengaged).

I suggest that the mapper could do a head count of the non-DCM participants in the room and mark them as engaged or disengaged at the beginning of each Time Frame. The mapper should only spend a few seconds observing each of the non-DCM participants. The grid on the bottom of the adapted raw data sheet should be used for this purpose. The mapper should record the number of people who are engaged and the number who are disengaged, because these will be needed to work out percentages later. As soon as a recording has been made of the level of engagement, the observations should then be carried out in the usual DCM methodology to collect WIB and BCC.

A worked data sheet is shown on the previous page. The WIB values would be calculated in the usual way. The percentage calculation is the percentage of non-DCM participants who were engaged. Therefore, first add up the total number of observations of non-DCM participants from the bottom row (10+10+ 12+...14+14). Put this figure in the bottom right-hand box (309 in this example). Then add together the number of participants engaged across all time frames (3+3+5+...2+2). Divide this figure (126) by the last calculation (309). Multiply by 100 to turn it into a percentage, rounding to the nearest whole number.

This provides us with the additional information that the rest of the residents who were not being mapped were engaged for approximately 41% of the time. This may equate to a WIB score of around +1, which is similar to those participants being mapped. Had this percentage been much higher than this it might have reflected that a lot of staff time was being spent with non-DCM participants. This might have meant that we were not getting a representative sample from the Dementia Care Map.

Conclusions

Combining DCM and Engagement in this way requires some extra field work and research. It is offered as a possible means of trying to enrich the DCM measure, which may be useful in some circumstances.

• Published in *JDC*, May/June 1999.

References

Bond S, Bond J (1990) Outcomes of care within a multiple-case study in the evaluation of the experimental National Health Service nursing homes. Age and Ageing 19 11-18.

Bradford Dementia Group (1997) Evaluating Dementia Care: The DCM Method. Seventh Edition. University of Bradford.

Brooker DJR (1994) Quality assurance – lessons learnt about putting it into practice. PSIGE (Psychologists Special Interest Group in the Elderly) Newsletter 48 37-41.

Brooker DJR, Dinshaw CJ (1998) A comparison of staff and patient feedback on mental health services for older people. Quality in Health Care 7 70-76.

Brooker DJR, Foster N, Banner A, Payne M, Jackson L (1998) Dementia Care Mapping: Report of Three Year British NHS Evaluation. Ageing and Mental Health 2 60 70.

Felce D, Powell L, Lunt , Jenkins J, Mansell J, (1980) Measuring activity of old people in residential care. Evaluation Review 4 371-387.

Godlove C, Richard L, Rodwell G (1982) Time for Action. Social Services Monograph: Research in Practice. Joint Unit for Social Services Research: Sheffield University .

Jenkins J, Felce D, Lunt B, Powell L (1977) Increasing engagement in activity of residents in old peoples homes by providing recreational materials. Behaviour Research and Therapy. 15, 429-434.

Kitwood T (1990) The dialectics of dementia: with particular reference to Alzheimer's disease. Ageing and Society 4 177-196.

Kitwood T, Bredin K (1992) A new approach to the evaluation of dementia care. Journal of Advances in Health and Nursing Care. 1 41-60.

McClannahan LE, Risley TR (1975) Design of living environments for nursing home residents: Increasing participation in recreation activities. Journal of Applied Behavior Analysis 8 261-268.

McCormack D, Whitehead A (1981) The effect of providing recreational activities on the engagement level of long-stay geriatric patients. Age and Ageing 10 287-291.

McFayden M (1984) The measurement of engagement in institutionalised elderly. In Hanley I, Hodge J (Eds) Psychological Approaches to Care of the Elderly. Croom Helm, London.

Nolan M, Grant G, Nolan J (1995) Busy doing nothing: activity and interaction levels amongst differing populations of elderly patients. Journal of Advanced Nursing 22 528-538.

23 Inter-rater reliability in Dementia Care Mapping

CLAIRE SURR, EVA BONDE NIELSEN

It is recommended during DCM training, that mappers work with at least with one other mapper during any DCM evaluation, as this offers them support throughout the process of briefing staff, analysing the data and feeding this back to staff. Since one mapper can only usually observe between 5 and 10 people, depending on their experience, teams of mappers are sometimes employed to ensure that as many people with dementia as possible, within in a care setting are mapped. When more than one observer will be conducting the mapping, or if mapping over time using different mappers (particularly in research and formal evaluations) it is important to consider the question of inter-rater reliability.

A NEW FORMAT FOR COMPARING DCM DATA FROM DIFFERENT MAPPERS TO MAKE IT EASIER TO IDENTIFY ANY DISCREPANCIES

Inter-rater reliability is a measure of how similar maps are between two mappers observing the same group of people at the same time. There will never be 100 per cent agreement between two mappers because DCM involves careful observation of signs of well-being and illbeing which are easy to miss on occasion. As a rule of thumb if there is about 70 per cent agreement between two mappers then this is taken as good enough to be relied upon in routine mapping. If DCM is being used in research it is recommended that the mapping team aim for 80 per cent agreement. There are a number of ways that inter-rater reliability in mapping can be improved upon.

Training in DCM

DCM is a complex tool. There are 24 possible behaviour category codes and up to six well- or ill-being values which may be chosen from for each five-minute observation period, for each person with dementia being mapped. The intensive three-day DCM (Basic) course, which is standardised in terms of content and teaching throughout the UK and worldwide, teaches course participants about coding and recognising levels of well and ill-being. Since people with dementia do not normally undertake just one type of behaviour within any five minute period, DCM employs some operational rules to help mappers to make a choice between categories, which are also taught on the basic course. Course participants are also required to achieve a minimum of 60 per cent on a written assessment to pass the basic course.

The more training a mapper undertakes in relation to the DCM method, and the greater the amount of mapping experience they have, the more reliable their mapping is likely to be in relation to the way the method is described in the manual, and to other experienced mappers. This was supported by an as yet unpublished study in Germany, conducted by Rusing (2003), who found reliability between two experienced mappers to be much higher (73 per cent) than reliability between an experienced mapper and a mapper who had just taken the basic DCM course (53 per cent). Therefore undertaking the DCM (Advanced) course during which participants receive further in depth instruction with regard to DCM coding, as well as addressing issues associated with implementing DCM in practice is likely to improve accuracy and reliability. Mappers who then go on to become DCM Evaluators and DCM trainers are likely to be more reliable still. However, the majority of mappers at present do not undertake further training in DCM following their basic course. There is also the issue that inter-rater reliability testing is not taught until the DCM Advanced course, however it is straightforward to conduct and is clearly set out in the DCM manual. Those having only taken DCM Basic training but who are mapping regularly should take time to learn this.

Testing for inter-rater reliability

Any mapper working alone or with other mappers therefore needs to consider their own standards of coding, and how they might upkeep or improve them. Conducting inter-rater reliability tests with other mappers are one way of doing this. To conduct an inter-rater reliability test two or more mappers observe the same people for a period of 1 hour. They then conduct a simple concordance coefficient calculation which is clearly set out in the DCM manual

There are a number of important issues for mappers to consider when conducting an inter-rater reliability test.
• Make sure that the inter-rater reliability test mapping is as similar to actual mapping as possible. If you regularly observe eight people with dementia then you should check your reliability under these conditions.
• Mappers need to consider how representative the reliability map they have conducted is in relation to the range of

BCCs and WIB values they are likely to code during the map itself. For example, if only five BCCs and two WIB values are observed in the reliability map, how sure can mappers be that they are reliable in coding the other BCCs and levels of well or ill being?

• When calculating the agreement scores mappers should examine every time frame when there was dis-agreement regarding a BCC or WIB and use their notes to discuss why this occurred. (For one suggested method for comparing data see below).

• They should consult the DCM manual and the operational rules to decide which code was correct. If they are still unsure they should consult a more experienced mapper locally, or the Bradford Dementia Group.

• If there is still not a good enough level of agreement mappers should discuss the differences and do a further reliability test until the appropriate level of agreement is achieved.

• Mappers should also look at the Personal Detractions (PDs) and Positive Events (PEs) they have coded during the reliability test, and compare these for the number recorded, type and level of severity of PDs, and the notes made concerning the incidents recorded. Accuracy between the mappers regarding the number of and types of incidents recorded should be aimed for.

• Mappers who are working alone within an organisation should aim to map and conduct an inter-rater reliability test with another, preferably more experienced mapper from outside their organisation at least once a year.

• Regional DCM network groups in the UK are one place links with other mappers can be formed (see the BDG website for details of a group in your region: www.brad.ac.uk/acad/health/bdg.htm).

• Mappers working together regularly run the risk of 'mapping drift', this is where they consistently code the same as other mappers within their organisation, but are not reliable with other mappers or the manual. Again mapping with more experienced mappers from other organisations can help to avoid this.

Current levels of inter-rater reliability are unknown, and we can assume that they will be fairly low where mappers are trained to the basic level, map infrequently, and do not conduct regular inter-rater reliability checks, and unpublished work by Thornton (cited by Fossey, 2001, p32-33) suggests that this is likely to be the case.

Comparing data

The DCM manual shows one format for comparing data from two mappers following a reliability test (see figure 1). However, one of the authors (Bonde Nielsen) has developed a format for comparing data in a slightly different way. This method makes it much easier to identify whether discrepancies in coding lie with coding behaviours, or well and ill-being, or both (see figure 2). This method can help to focus mappers onto the areas where there are differences. It does not matter which method mappers use to compare their inter-rater reliability data, what is important is that inter-rater reliability tests are conducted regularly, and that discrepancies in coding are discussed.

Participant Name (Peter J)	Time	10 00	10 05	10 10	10 15	10 20	10 25	10 30	10 35	10 40	10 45	10 50	10 55
Observer 1 (KD)	BCC	F	F	B	B	N	B	C	B	J	J	B	A
	WIB	+1	+3	+1	+1	+1	+1	-1	+1	+3	+3	+1	+3
Observer 2 (PT)	BCC	F	F	F	B	N	N	C	C	J	J	B	A
	WIB	+1	+1	+1	+1	+1	+1	-1	-1	+1	+3	+1	+3
Agreement		2	1	1	2	2	1	2	0	1	2	2	2

Figure 1 – Comparing data for Inter-rater Reliability Testing as in DCM Manual. Reliability for Peter J = 18/24 = 0.75 or 75%

	10 00	10 05	10 10	10 15	10 20	10 25	10 30	10 35	10 40	10 45	10 50	10 55
+5												
+3	F								J	JJ		AA
+1	FF	F	BF	BB	NN	BN		B	J		BB	
-1							CC	C				
-3												
-5												
	2	1	1	2	2	1	2	0	1	2	2	2

Figure 2 – An Alternative Way of Comparing DCM Data for Inter-rater Reliability Testing. **BOLD** = Observer 1. **LIGHT** = Observer 2. Presenting the data from two observers immediately highlights which BCCs and WiB values are being coded differently.

**Claire's personal experience
of mapping across cultures**

On a personal level I found mapping in Denmark only a little more difficult than mapping in the UK in terms of assigning codes. The problems arose, however, when participants spoke to me, when Eva was introducing us to the group on arrival, during the mapping and again when we thanked people before we left. I was not able to understand what was being said to me, nor to be sure that I was responding appropriately. I did smile, shake hands with people and use appropriate body language, but I was still left feeling uncomfortable about not being able to communicate back effectively. I feel the way we as mappers communicate with the people with dementia we are mapping is an issue for all mappers to consider; communication skills may not be simply transferable to another country.

Reliability across cultures

Since there are now DCM trained personnel throughout the world, and training is available through strategic partnerships in five other countries at present, issues relating to inter-rater reliability within and across different cultures are also highly relevant. Therefore while Claire Surr was on a recent visit to Denmark, she and Eva Bonde Neilsen decided to use the opportunity conduct an inter-rater reliability map.

We visited a care facility in Copenhagen where mapping regularly takes place, and is part of the ongoing quality checking and improvement mechanisms of the facility. Both the staff and residents were used to mappers being present on a regular basis. We conducted the map in the day centre unit, where there were seven people with dementia (participants) present and three members of staff. All the participants were mobile, and had varying levels of dementia. We both mapped five participants for two hours, and throughout this time no English was spoken. Since Claire does not speak Danish, this proved an interesting exercise. All she had to go on with regard to coding both behaviours and levels of well or ill-being was actions, body language, facial expressions and tone of voice.

Overall, however, we achieved a concordance coefficient of 92 per cent, agreeing on 180 out of 196 observations. The lowest reliability we achieved on an individual level was 88 per cent and the highest 95 per cent. Overall we observed participants engaged in 14 different behaviours including interaction (A), singing (E), eating and drinking (F), handicrafts (H), participating in a quiz (I) and peeling potatoes for lunch (L). However, since the facility was offering care of a very high standard, we coded only positive WIB values (+1, +3 and +5) and did not observe any ill-being. Therefore we cannot assume reliability in coding ill-being between the two mappers.

Although there were few disagreements the majority of these came on the ratings of well and ill-being. In most cases this related to Eva assigning a higher level of well-being than Claire had, as the context of people's conversa-tions indicated this higher level, for example if a person was engaged in very personal reminiscences, which Claire could not understand. However, we feel that from the limited data we have, we can assume that a high level of inter-rater reliability is possible, even across cultures and when the mappers cannot necessarily understand the communications of the participants.

Conclusion

Improving inter-rater reliability between mappers is an issue being considered further by Bradford Dementia Group, and we are keen in the future to develop multiple ways of doing this – for example through putting video clips on the web for mappers to code, developing a network of 'Gold Standard' mappers throughout the UK and worldwide, and holding coding refresher sessions as part of the regional network groups. There is currently an international working group examining issues of reliability and validity of DCM for the purposes of improving this for the DCM 8th edition of the method, due for launch in 2005. However, in addition to this it remains important that all mappers continue to conduct inter-rater reliability checks on a regular basis, and aim to map with more experienced mappers whenever possible.

• Published in *JDC*, Nov/Dec 2003.

Bibliography

Ballard C, Fossey J, Chithramohan R, Howard R, Burns A, Thompson P, Tadros G, Fairburn A (2001) Quality of Care in Private Sector and NHS Facilities for People with Dementia: Cross Sectional Survey. *British Medical Journal* 323 426-7.

Bradford Dementia Group (1997) *Evaluating Dementia Care. The DCM Method* 7th Edition. University of Bradford.

Brooker D (2001) Enriching Lives: Evaluation of the ExtraCare Activity Challenge. *Journal Of Dementia Care* 9(3) 33-37.

Brooker D, Duce L (2000) Wellbeing and Activity in Dementia: A Comparison of Group Reminiscence Therapy, Structured Goal-Directed Group Activity and Unstructured Time. *Aging and Mental Health* 4(4) 354-358.

Brooker D, Foster J, Banner A, Payne M, Jackson L (1998) The Efficacy of Dementia Care Mapping as an Audit Tool: Report of a 3-Year British NHS Evaluation. *Aging and Mental Health* 2(1) 60-70.

Fossey J (2001) In what ways does DCM need to be modified in order to maximise its usefulness in promoting improvements in the quality of life and quality of care for people with dementia? In Brooker D, Rogers L (Eds) *Dementia Care Mapping Think Tank Transcripts*. Bradford Dementia Group.

Jacques I (1996) Evaluating Care Services for People living with Dementia. *Elderly Care* 8(3) 10-13.

Kuhn D, Kasayka RE, Lechner C (2002) Behavioural Observations and Quality of life Among Persons with Dementia in 10 Assisted Living Facilities. *American Journal of Alzheimer's Disease and Other Dementias* 17(5) 291-298.

Martin GW, Younger D (2001) Person-centred Care for People with Dementia: A Quality Audit Approach. *Journal of Psychiatric and Mental Health Nursing* 8 443-448.

Rusing D (2003) Possible Statistics for DCM Coding. Unpublished paper.

24 DCM training – three or five days?

PAUL EDWARDS

One of the constant challenges to DCM trainers is being able to provide an in-depth training course on the method of DCM and its philosophy within three days. Course participants over many years have been consistent in evaluating the course positively but a large proportion of them have suggested that the course needed to be longer to allow for greater time to become confident in using the method.

EXPERIENCES OF RUNNING A FIVE-DAY DCM COURSE IN CHARNWOOD AND NORTH WEST LEICESTERSHIRE PRIMARY CARE TRUST

Historically an extended course of four or five days has not been an option largely due to the increased costs this would entail. However, over the last two years I have been fortunate to be able to pilot a five-day DCM course within an organisation. The course covers the same content as the first three days of any DCM course but the fourth and fifth days include actual practice mapping in 'real' environments and also allow for mappers to run briefing and feedback sessions to direct caregivers in those practice areas.

The idea behind this is to take mapping from the classroom into care areas in a safe and supportive way. New mappers are encouraged to use their skills and receive the advice of more experienced mappers who will guide and assist.

On the five-day DCM training course, course participants go out to a clinical area and brief care staff about mapping. Care staff are then asked to complete a feedback sheet that is shared with the course participants following the 1-2 hour practice maps on the area. Following mapping the data is brought back and analysed with trainers and then developed into preliminary feedback. This data is then presented back to the care team on the next day and again care teams are asked to complete a short questionnaire on how the data was fed back by the course participants.

At first read this may sound a scary addition to an already intensive course, but all the mappers I have trained in this way have welcomed the option of actually mapping in a safe learning environment. Basic users who complete the three-day course can leave feeling very apprehensive about completing their first map. Also if there is no one else around within their organisation with experience of mapping then it can be quite a hurdle trying to achieve a first map with some confidence.

Setting up a five-day DCM course

Careful planning is a crucial part of any DCM course but with extra days that include practice maps and briefing and feedback to real care teams, it requires particular attention. The central consideration has to be the organisation hosting the course. The host organisation needs to have had many opportunities to discuss the process and ideally needs to have DCM established. There should be strong lines of communication between trainers and all levels of the organisation and clear 'up front' discussions should be held detailing the benefits and problems with extending the training course. Care teams need to be fully briefed and supported as they play a key role in providing feedback to the new basic users. At every level there should be inclusion. Safeguards such as having experienced users of the method on hand during the briefing, practice and feedback need to be in place and clinical areas should know whom they can turn to if there are any problems.

Careful consideration needs to be made to the logistics of having new users practising across different sites. For every practice mapping area there needs to be a 'buddy' for both the mappers and the care teams. Having more experienced users around at the time of the briefing, mapping and feedback allows for any difficulties to be quickly rectified for mappers and care teams alike. This is reassuring for all concerned and also promotes a spirit of joint learning and collaboration.

It is also important that course participants have the chance to de-brief following their mapping experience. It seems to be in the nature of DCM that it unlocks a whole new window on the world of caring. Often course participants will not necessarily be used to observing for long periods of time and this can be a challenge to the hearts and minds of mappers. Much care and attention to the pastoral needs of participants at this time of the course is essential. On one of my courses a new user observed a 'degeneration run' for one participant who appeared withdrawn for over an hour with no contact from anyone. This greatly affected her and she needed time to talk it through in a safe way with other users and trainers. She also needed support as during the mapping she did make contact with the person and felt she'd 'done the wrong thing in DCM terms' as she'd moved from observer to care giver. Once she received the support and advice she needed she was able to go back the next day and give feedback.

The Course Structure

The course mirrors the three-day DCM basic course. During the first three days participants learn about the background and structure of DCM and also the underpinning philosophy of person-centred care. Participants learn about the application of DCM and undertake an assessment. On the afternoon of the third day, greater depth about briefing and feedback is given and also the logistical arrangements are made.

On the fourth day all course participants brief a care team for around 15 minutes and then undertake around 1.5 hours' mapping. That data is then brought back and analysed and participants are guided through the process of how to write and present such items as individual care summaries and WIB and behaviour profiles. It needs to be stressed that we are only working with small amounts of data on an individual and this is merely a practice, although care teams have said they have learnt something from even this small amount of data during the course of these practice maps.

Feedback is given to the care team on the fifth day and again this needs intensive support for teams and mappers alike. The participants on the last two five-day courses rate this part as even more anxiety provoking than the assessment on day three! New users, though, identify how important this is once they have delivered the feedback.

Evaluation of the five-day training

The five-day course, just like the three-day course, has been received very well by its participants. Like the three-day course many participants have found it intensive, motivating and relevant.

Where the evaluations differ is in the experience of providing 'real' practice at mapping. All participants appreciate this opportunity to map in a supported way and all evaluations reflect a greater confidence in the use of the tool. Participants indicated that the briefing and feedback sessions with actual ward teams and actual data was beneficial to their experience. The feedback they received from the care teams was positive and all participants felt they could learn something about the process of mapping from the two days of practice.

A few participants felt as if they had been on an emotional roller coaster for the whole week and there were some examples on the evaluation forms depicting the journey that some had travelled. One wrote:

It has been a roller-coaster of a course – with high anxiety, great fun and serious reflections. I felt uncomfortable about having to brief and give feedback on wards that I knew, but it was a really worthwhile part of the course. I felt emotionally drained now but confident that I can map again with some skill.

A simple inter-rater reliability check of the new mappers was also conducted. The range across the five different teams was 68% (lowest) and 91% (highest). This again could be discussed with the participants and having the extra two days allowed us to reinforce issues about applying the tool.

Lessons learnt

The five-day course does offer the participant the chance to practise DCM in a supported way. It does allow new users of the tool to gain experience and confidence. It also consolidates theory.

For a five-day course to work in this way a strong commitment has to be made by the organisation running it. There are more initial costs involved, as staff have to be released for longer. Clinical areas will need to cover shifts and also the extra costs of freeing up more experienced users to support the practical experience. This is justified, though, as people leave the five-day course with a unique experience and are more motivated to make DCM work within the organisation.

This course ideally needs to be run in an organisation that has a strong commitment to person-centred care and has experienced mappers within it who can support clinical areas during the last two days.

The organisation will already have strong developmental structures supporting DCM and will need a clear vision. Providing that this is the backdrop to the five-day course, the real benefits of running a longer DCM course are obvious. Of course having confident and motivated mappers is essential but more than this, it allows members of care teams not attending the course to be part of the learning. Their feedback to the new users of the method helps with relationships and reduces the mystery of the process of DCM. When this happens DCM is more likely to be an accepted part of practice.

As a trainer it is always rewarding seeing people leave a DCM course with motivation, energy and a greater understanding of how we can improve care for people with dementia. With the five-day course something unique happens; as a trainer you get to 'roll your sleeves up' and map alongside course participants. Issues about applying DCM can be quickly resolved and this is done as an integral part of the learning process on a course. Participants who have undertaken this course leave with a skill they can be more confident about and this ultimately bodes well for the organisation. It is easier to make DCM a reality within an organisation if mappers are confident and experienced. There is a very strong argument that a five-day course enables the transition of knowledge from theory into practice in a hugely rewarding way for the host organisation, the course participant and the trainer.

• Published in JDC, Jan/Feb 2004.

Before and after training: a case study of intervention

25

TRACEY LINTERN, BOB WOODS, LYNNE PHAIR

In 1994 the late Tom Kitwood was commissioned with one of us (BW) to produce a document outlining a staff training and development strategy for RSAS AgeCare. This set out 'best practice' in relation to the charity's new nursing home, which was to have a significant dementia care component (Kitwood & Woods 1995). As envisaged in the strategy document, the action research programme to be described in this series of articles was then undertaken. The aim was to evaluate the extent to which staff training and development would improve resident well-being and quality of life.

The assumption underlying the project is that training and development will impact on staff attitudes and beliefs, knowledge and skills, so that the behaviour and interactions of staff with residents will change and have an effect on residents' quality of life. In evaluating this process, it was important to assess changes in staff as well as in residents. To do this, it was necessary to develop a battery of assessments, the Dementia Care Practitioner Assessment (DCPA - Lintern & Woods 1996), which together provide an indication of staff attitudes, knowledge and skills. The components of the DCPA include the following:

• Attitudes to people with dementia: assessed by the 19-item Approaches to Dementia Questionnaire (ADQ) and the Dementia Care Styles Questionnaire (DCS - Brooker et al, 1998).

• Knowledge about dementia: assessed using a multiple-choice dementia quiz adapted from Gilleard & Groom (1994).

• Response to video scenarios: staff are asked to report their reactions to 11 'typical' brief scenes from daily life in a home; in some the task is to identify negative and positive aspects of the interactions shown, in others suggestions are invited as to how to tackle the potentially difficult situation depicted. Responses are coded to indicate the types of needs identified by the staff member and their approaches to problem solving.

• Observations of staff behaviour: most observational methods focus on the resident, whereas in DCPA it is the staff member's input to the observed interactions which is coded. The amount and type of contact staff have with residents is noted, and the way in which physical care is provided is

> **CAN STAFF TRAINING AND DEVELOPMENT IMPROVE RESIDENTS' WELL-BEING? THIS CHAPTER DESCRIBES A RESEARCH PROJECT IN A NURSING HOME**

evaluated. Observations take place only in communal areas of the dementia care unit, to respect residents' privacy.

The main outcome measure for resident well being and quality of life used in the project was the Dementia Care Mapping methodology developed by Kitwood and colleagues at the Bradford Dementia Group. It is debatable to what extent DCM is a measure of quality of care rather than of quality of life, but we would contend that in a residential context the two domains may converge, with much of quality of life dependent upon the quality of care inputs provided.

An overview of the home

The project began in June 1996, just over a year after the first residents were admitted. The home is purpose-built, with 50 beds, excellent facilities and an award-winning design. The building is separated into two units, one for elderly people with physical frailties and the other for elderly people with dementia. Both units are further split into two 'villages' with between 12 and 14 residents each. The units are separated by a large concourse area where functions, activities, fêtes and tea parties are held. There are a number of homely styled communal lounges and 'quiet rooms' in each village and a number of large well-equipped bathrooms and toilets. All residents have their own single room where they may have their own furniture and possessions. There are well-kept, safely fenced gardens and patio areas accessible from the main lounges. The home is tastefully furnished and decorated with high standards of cleanliness being maintained.

At baseline, there were approximately 44 residents (10-12 in each village) ranging in age from 65-100 years. The staff group consisted of 34 care assistants (including 15 night staff), none of whom had received any formal training in caring for elderly people or for people with dementia. Approximately 70 per cent of the care assistants had some previous experience of working with elderly people. There were also 9 RGNs [1] (including 3 night staff), 6 RMNs [2] (including 2 night staff) and 1 EN [3]. The average resident to staff ratio was 4 or 5:1 on each village per shift. The day

[1] RGN – Registered General Nurse; [2] RMN – Registered Mental Nurse; [3] EN – Enrolled Nurse

staff worked either an early shift (8am to 2.15pm) or a late shift (2.15pm to 8.30pm). They were also frequently asked to work a 'long day' – a 12.5-hour shift from 8am to 8.30pm, and would sometimes work up to six of these in a row.

A rotational system was in place for staff whereby care assistants worked in two groups, one group working with residents who have dementia, and the other with physically frail residents in the other unit. Every four weeks the two groups of staff (with the exception of qualified staff) swapped units, although in view of the difficulty in recruiting RMNs, RGNs also had to work on both units. Most care assistants reported that they liked working in this way as it introduced variety to their work and they appreciated 'having a break' from working in one unit all the time. However, this system clearly had implications for the continuity of care for residents and, perhaps more importantly, constrained the development of meaningful relationships between care staff and residents. Such a system may encourage staff to remain distant from those in their care, since they work with them for only four weeks and then move on.

During the baseline period, it became clear from interviews and observations that a number of aspects of the suggested strategy had yet to be implemented:
• The senior care staff had not received training in supervision and no supervision mechanisms had been put in place
• An adequate induction programme for direct care staff was not in place
• Appropriate record-keeping reflecting the full range of experience of residents including some life history and positive care planning was minimal
• There was no key worker or primary nurse system
• There were no arrangements for in-service training.

Staff/resident interaction

The organisation of staff was clearly hierarchical, with care assistants given little opportunity to contribute their opinions or experiences, or be involved in decision making. Staff meetings occurred infrequently, were problem-focused and did not appear to facilitate an open exchange of views and ideas between all levels of staff. Shift handovers occurred between the two qualified members of staff in charge, while care assistants immediately began direct care work. Therefore little information about previous shifts, the well being of the residents or information about any new residents admitted was communicated to care assistants coming on duty.

The initial research interviews also indicated that many care assistants were concerned about the absence of any induction training and the lack of feedback received about their work and progress. They conveyed the impression of a group which was somewhat uncertain about the direction and appropriateness of its work.

During the initial Dementia Care Mapping evaluation it was noticeable that interaction between staff and residents was limited with a focus primarily on the physical care of residents to the exclusion of their psychological needs. Residents frequently expressed anxiety or distress to which staff did not respond. Interviews indicated that this was because staff attributed symptoms of anxiety and distress to the resident's medical condition which therefore could not be helped.

Significant emphasis was placed on the appearance of both the environment and the residents. For example, an interior decorator was employed to provide a tasteful and homely atmosphere to the building; staff prided themselves on the level of cleanliness and hygiene within the home and were frequently observed tidying and spraying air freshener; and every effort was made to ensure that residents' hair was always tidy and their clothes clean and colour co-ordinated.

Few activities, events or daily tasks for the benefit of the residents were observed during the first six months of the project. Some events including tea parties, sing-songs and the occasional entertainment by a pianist, organist, theatre group or choir were organised by the home's 'Friends'. A gentle exercise session and an art class also occurred once a week, attended mainly by residents from the physically frail unit; residents with dementia were given little opportunity to participate.

A culture had developed whereby responsibility for organising activities was handed over to outside agencies, rather than one where purposeful activity is considered part of the daily care. On occasions, staff were observed providing some stimulation for residents, but their approach was not personalised, in terms of the individual resident's background, preferences or abilities. For example, they may have been handed a book to read or look at alone, taken for a short walk around the garden, or encouraged to watch television.

There was little scope for residents to become involved in domestic activities and many 'missed opportunities' were observed where an attempt by a resident to do something constructive was thwarted by carers offering to do it for them. This was undoubtedly well-intentioned on the part of staff who perceived that their role was to 'look after' the home and the residents and were clearly trying to be helpful.

Provision for residents to retain a measure of control over their daily lives appeared limited: for example, 'toilet rounds' and a bath rota were employed at times convenient for the staff rather than the personal preference of the resident.

During this initial phase, several points of basic safety awareness were noted. On occasion, for instance, wheelchairs were tipped backwards with the residents in them and pushed along on the back wheels, rather than using foot-plates for their usual purpose. Once brought to the attention of the home manager, this practice was curtailed. The recognition of residents' risk of falling and the taking of appropriate precautionary measures was problematic at times. Attempts to provide for the need of some residents to walk and exercise safely were not always present. Residents at risk of falling were frequently told to sit down and were put back in a chair by staff each time they tried to stand up. On occasions, the positioning of furniture led to a great deal of frustration, anger and distress on the part of such residents. Incidents observed during DCM indicated that interventions were required to help staff consider the resident's perspective in effectively assessing potential risks and in developing appropriate preventive actions.

The first intervention

The first intervention consisted of a two day training course for the home's senior staff (heads of care and manager) followed by a two-day training course for direct care staff. The training focused on developing person-centred dementia care and was facilitated by Dr Tom Kitwood of the Bradford Dementia Group. Specifically, it consisted of the following elements:

Senior managers

Training days with senior staff concentrated on the extent to which the objectives of the Training and Development Strategy had been applied, with discussion of areas in need of development and direction. A development plan was constructed including the following points:

- Establishment of a supervision protocol
- An overhaul of the personnel interview techniques
- Development of induction procedures
- Development of life history documentation
- Development of care planning practices
- Establishment of a key worker system
- Establishment of a programme of ongoing in-house training

- Development of the involvement of relatives in the home.

Care staff: groups 1 and 2

The two-day training for care staff used a range of techniques, including traditional lecturing, interactive discussions, role-play demonstrations and small group work to explore a number of issues. Specifically, areas of focus included:

- Exploring differences between 'old and new cultures of care' and reflecting upon where the home was positioned in this regard
- Understanding the concept of an individual's unique personhood and reflecting on experiences where one's own personhood had and had not been respected
- Demonstration and discussion of the malignant social psychology of dementia care
- Explanation and exercise in dementia care mapping (DCM) and outline of the home's DCM results
- Dramatised demonstration of the importance of life history and exercise in appreciating the uniqueness of individuals
- A group exercise to explore methods of communication of people with dementia and understanding the meaning of such communication
- Understanding the psychological needs of people with dementia
- Reflecting on practice.

The sessions were interactive with participants being given the opportunity to ask questions, discuss issues and raise particular difficulties. Following the two training days, some members of staff completed projects designed to develop a more individualised approach which enabled them to receive certificates of attendance with assessment from Bradford University. Half the staff were trained at a time, with an interval of three months between the first and second staff groups receiving training.

Results of the intervention

Responses to the questionnaires indicated that staff chose significantly more person-centred responses and fewer disease-focused ones when asked how they would respond to certain situations. The ADQ indicated a more hopeful attitude to people with dementia among the staff. In particular, staff were less likely to agree with statements suggesting (a) that people with dementia are very much like children, (b) are

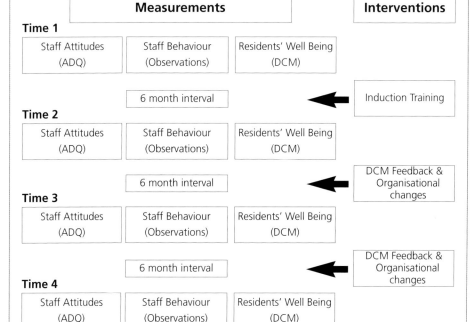

unable to make decisions, (c) will inevitably go downhill and (d) that it is important not to become too attached to residents.

Responses to the video vignettes indicated that staff were significantly more aware of residents' needs for independence, occupation, understanding and self worth and were less likely to focus on the neatness of the environment. They also indicated that they were more likely to use problem solving strategies in responding to residents.

Observations indicated that following training staff engaged in activities and social interactions with residents significantly more than previously; their interactions during physical care were of significantly higher quality; and they made significantly fewer remarks that could undermine or devalue residents.

Disappointingly however, the second DCM evaluation indicated little change had occurred since the last evaluation, with positive changes in overall scores only being seen on one of the villages. Here, the overall distribution of well-being values shifted upwards significantly, suggesting that there was a greater proportion of more positively-rated care episodes. There was no significant improvement in the average well-being scores of individual residents.

Because the training for care staff was delivered to care staff in two groups, three months apart, the opportunity arose to readminister the ADQ, DCS questionnaire and Dementia Quiz to both groups just before the second group received their training, so that they served as a control group for comparison purposes. There were no significant differences between groups on these measures, suggesting the effects of training were not specific to those attending. This would be a positive finding, if training one group of staff were changing the culture of care; however, it fails to confirm that any changes are directly attributable to the training and not to other influences.

At this point in the project, we had not yet been able to demonstrate a positive change in resident well being. However, an encouraging number of positive and potentially important changes in staff attitudes, skills and behaviour were evident following the initial two-day training intervention. In Chapter 26 we will look at the further work which was needed in order to develop these staff changes into positive outcomes for residents.

References

Brooker D, Foster N, Banner A, Payne M & Jackson L (1998). The efficacy of Dementia Care Mapping as an audit tool: report of a 3-year British NHS evaluation. *Aging & Mental Health* 2 60-70.

Gilleard C & Groom F (1994). A study of two dementia quizzes. British Journal of Clinical Psychology, 33, 529-534.

Kitwood T & Woods RT (1995). *A training and development strategy for dementia care in residential settings*. Bradford Dementia Group, Bradford.

Lintern T, Woods RT (1996). The Dementia Care Practitioner Assessment (DCPA). *Baseline - Journal of the British Association for Service to the Elderly* 63 12-18.

Acknowledgement

We are most grateful to: RSAS AgeCare for funding this project; staff and residents of the Bradbury Centre; Elizabeth Barnett for assistance with DCM; and of course the late Tom Kitwood for inspiration.

• Published in *JDC*, Jan/Feb 2000.

26 Training is not enough to change care practice

TRACEY LINTERN, BOB WOODS, LYNNE PHAIR

In Chapter 25, we described the first phase of a training and development programme, in a newly opened 50-bed nursing home. Two of the home's four "villages" were specifically for people with dementia, and these were the focus of this action research project. All staff participated in two days' training in person-centred dementia care with the late Tom Kitwood of the Bradford Dementia Group.

There were a number of positive changes in staff attitudes and in the interactions of staff with residents, measured using the Dementia Care Practitioner Assessment (DCPA). However, the impact on residents' well-being, assessed using Dementia Care Mapping (DCM), was limited. In one village, there was a significant shift with more episodes of care being rated positively, but the well-being scores of individual residents did not show an improvement immediately following training. In this article we describe the process of translating changes in staff attitudes and behaviour into improved well-being for the residents in their care.

The second intervention phase

The major intervention during this six-month period was based around the feedback to staff from the DCM carried out after the training sessions had been completed. For various practical reasons, the feedback sessions took place several months after the actual evaluation had taken place. An action plan was drawn up with the staff group, arising from issues identified in the feedback. It addressed a number of developmental and organisational issues, which were supported by a new home manager with a keen commitment to person-centred care, and extended further by a newly appointed senior nurse, with responsibilities for quality across all of the RSAS AgeCare homes (LP).

Action plan
The following objectives were established:
• Staff would seek to reduce the number of personal detractions, including discussing residents in their presence. For example, handovers would no longer occur in the lounge areas
• Staff would try to engage residents in more activities; to

> HOW CAN CHANGES IN STAFF ATTITUDES AND BEHAVIOUR BE TRANSLATED INTO IMPROVED WELL-BEING FOR NURSING HOME RESIDENTS?

promote this, the manager would buy more activity equipment
• Staff would attempt to give more attention to residents who were less able to express their needs, and had tended to be relatively neglected
• The head of care would develop personal profiles for all residents to which care staff and relatives could contribute
• More attention would be paid to residents who slept a great deal and attempts made to include them in unit activities wherever possible
• Staff would attempt to facilitate residents who wished to walk or wander
• Staff would attempt to pay more attention to residents in distress and attempt to understand what they were trying to communicate
• The monthly rotation of staff between the dementia care unit and the physically frail unit would be phased out, with staff having as much choice as possible regarding their placement
• Supervision and support of senior managers: there was no provision for supervision in the home. In order to begin introducing this in the home and to provide guidance and support to senior staff, the manager and heads of care underwent an intensive period of supervisory sessions with the senior nurse
• Appointment of a part-time nurse development practitioner: many of the care assistants reported feeling that they did not receive enough leadership and direction from the senior members of staff. This problem could potentially have limited the impact of the initial training input, particularly if the efforts of staff were not being reinforced and encouraged in practice by senior role models on a regular basis. In order to develop this area, leadership responsibilities were clarified and an additional member of staff was employed to work with care assistants for two days a week, providing guidance as a professional role model as well as providing hands-on training, and facilitating more formal training through induction manuals and National Vocational Qualifications.

Changes after second intervention

DCPA Questionnaires: Responses to the questionnaires indicated that, since the last evaluation, staff were choosing significantly more person-centred responses, and fewer behavioural and normalising responses when asked how they would respond to certain situations. The attitude scale indicated significantly more positive general attitudes and in particular, it again showed a significant increase in level of hopefulness among staff.

DCPA Videos: Responses to the video vignettes indicated further significant increases in staff awareness of the residents' need for occupation. No significant differences were found in the strategies suggested for responding to residents.

DCPA Observations: Observations of staff indicated that there had been further significant increases in the amount of time spent engaged in activities with residents. There were also significantly more physical care interactions.

Dementia Care Mapping: The third DCM evaluation indicated significant positive changes in care values ▮ had occurred since the last evaluation, with improvements being seen in both dementia care villages. As before, no significant change in individual resident well-being scores were noted.

The third intervention phase

The intervention during this period again consisted of an action plan formulated from the observations made during the DCM evaluation, but on this occasion the feedback was given less than a week after the observation period. It was anticipated that this would have a greater impact on the staff. The issues raised would be more pertinent – being more easily able to recall the events that occurred during observation, staff would be more likely to accept the results as valid and commit themselves to making the necessary changes.

Action plan

Following the feedback session, the development plan drawn up included the following objectives:
• To increase the variety of physical activity available to residents; for example, by encouraging them to work with staff on chores as well as more structured "games"
• To increase residents' intellectual stimulation; for example, by purchasing more appropriate puzzles than those presently available
• To increase sensory stimulation for residents, particularly those with low physical and verbal abilities
• To encourage independence of residents who enjoy walking by keeping doors open during good weather rather than encouraging them to sit down or locking/blocking the doors
• To utilise "spare" time before lunch for purposeful activity
• To give residents appropriate cues at lunch times, for example by laying tables and helping them to their seats not more than 10 minutes before lunch arrives, and by

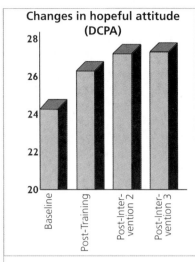

Changes in hopeful attitude (DCPA)

(bars labelled: Baseline, Post-Training, Post-Intervention 2, Post-Intervention 3; y-axis 20 to 28)

encouraging residents who are willing and able to help with preparations – by laying the tables, for example
• To communicate the home's philosophy to bank and agency staff in order to maintain continuity of care even in periods of staff shortage
• To introduce an overlap time between shifts (30 minutes morning and evening; 1 hour in the afternoon), so that all members of the incoming shift could attend handovers. As noted in the previous article, handovers previously included only the two qualified members of staff in charge, hampering communication and planning of care. Some of the overlap time was now also earmarked for further staff development, such as staff training or group supervision sessions, or for addressing specific issues of care and discussions of particular residents
• To introduce an induction programme for new members of qualified staff focusing on person-centred care, with a view to extending the programme to new members of the care staff. The initial focus was on qualified staff, as it was clear that the effectiveness of care staff training was essentially reliant on the ability of those in charge of the day-to-day running of the shifts to implement any necessary changes. If junior staff were receiving mixed messages about issues of good practice, then this could potentially inhibit progress towards higher quality care
• To replace the rather clinical uniforms that were in use in the home with a neat but more casual dress code. This was in order to create a more relaxed and homely environment
• To extend the garden fence: during DCM feedback, staff concerns regarding the frustration of residents at having limited space in which to walk were discussed. Extending the fence would provide a greater sense of freedom and satisfaction for residents.
• To disconnect the exit alarm: this system was intended to warn staff of a resident leaving the village, but, during DCM feedback, the almost continual bleeping noise emitted was identified as a major factor in creating an unsettling atmosphere. In its place, staff agreed to allocate someone to monitor those residents who were particularly vulnerable.

Changes after third intervention

DCPA Questionnaires: No further significant changes were indicated by the questionnaires at this time.
DCPA Videos: Responses to the video vignettes indicated

▮ Care values – the equivalent of WIB values in the 6th edition of DCM further significant increases in staff awareness of the residents need for self worth. No significant differences were found in the strategies suggested for responding to residents.

DCPA Observations: No further significant changes were indicated.

Dementia Care Mapping: The fourth DCM evaluation indicated yet further positive change had occurred since the last evaluation. Again the proportion of WiB values shifted to become more positive, and now, compared with baseline and the post-training evaluation, there was a significant improvement in the average individual resident's well-being. This could not be attributed to changes in functional disability of the residents on the unit, as there were no differences over the course of the project on any of the sub-scales of the behaviour rating scale used regularly on the unit (Ward et al, 1991). By this stage, the number of personal detractions (statements or actions which restrict or devalue) made were greatly reduced (almost to nil).

What the results showed

The results of the project indicate that while most of the changes in staff attitude and behaviour were evident after the initial training phase, it was only after two further six-month periods of developmental change, based on DCM feedback to staff, that improvements in resident well-being could be demonstrated (see graphs).

By this time, some considerable developmental progress had been achieved at the home. Staff now worked regular shifts with overlap times for handovers which greatly enhanced communication with each other. Staff now had one unit with which they could identify, enhancing greatly stability, continuity of care, the development of relationships between staff and residents, and a sense of team cohesion. Communication among the staff had also been assisted by the introduction of more regular team meetings and senior staff meetings focusing on growth and development, balanced with praise and guidance.

There was also a much greater awareness among staff of the necessity for psychological care alongside physical care, with a holistic, individualised approach being favoured. Residents were now given more choice, more freedom, more opportunities to remain active and to express themselves and a more relaxed and stable environment. Early concerns about the safety of residents were readily addressed and strategies put in place to ensure that all staff were aware of and updated on manual handling procedures and that particularly vulnerable residents were closely monitored. Induction programs were initiated for new staff and the opportunity provided for care assistants to work towards National Vocation Qualifications (NVQs).

Although these considerable achievements were accomplished by the combined efforts of many of the home's staff and associates, there were still a number of aspects from the Training and Development Strategy (Kitwood & Woods,

1995) that remained undeveloped. For example, further training was planned for qualified staff so that they would be in a better position to provide supervision and guidance for other staff. Similarly, a primary nurse system had been introduced, but further training would contribute to a more effective use of this system. Record keeping with regard to residents underwent some scrutiny and the manner in which care plans and personal profiles were maintained was thought to be maturing. There was, however, still opportunity to make more effective use of such documents. Finally, the provision of in-house training had clearly progressed, particularly for qualified staff and new staff; if this were extended to all staff (including domestic and support staff) it would constitute a comprehensive programme.

While such measures are likely to enhance and encourage good practice in the home, they can only really be implemented by a skilled and cohesive senior staff team and difficulties in recruiting and retaining suitable qualified nurses may well have restricted progression in some of these areas. In order to address this, a number of measures were planned, including an in-house training programme to develop the leadership skills of the existing qualified nurses.

Conclusions drawn from the process

This has been the story of one home, equipped with excellent physical facilities, which despite intending to be "person-centred" from the outset, took several years from its opening to reach a point where the well-being of people with dementia was being addressed adequately. What can other homes and organisations learn from our action research project?

1) Training alone did not lead to improved outcomes for residents, although it did appear to be related to changes in staff attitudes and behaviour that may underpin such outcomes later

2) Improved attitudes and skills shown by staff may not be sufficient to produce good outcomes for residents where there are organisational obstacles holding back positive change. These also must be addressed

3) Feedback needs to be timely for maximum effectiveness; the third intervention appeared to be more powerful than the second, where feedback was delayed

4) Measures of staff competence, such as the DCPA, may be especially useful in assisting with the evaluation of staff training, picking up changes earlier than measures such as DCM, which may be dependent additionally on changes in the residents' functional ability and health. (For further details of the availability of the DCPA, please contact Bob Woods.)

There is remarkably little evidence that training of staff in dementia care makes a difference to the residents in their care (Burgio & Burgio 1990). Our experience suggests that without attention to the organisational and management context in which the training takes place, the potential effectiveness of training inputs may often be diminished. There is, in our view, little purpose to be served in sending staff on training courses and/or organising in-house training sessions, if there is not the determination and will at a management and organisational level to overcome barriers to individualized, person-centred care. Such care requires good communication between staff in order to plan and implement care sensitively, and good two-way communication between management and staff, in order to reinforce and support staff in implementing this challenging, but ultimately rewarding, philosophy of care.

References

Burgio LD & Burgio KL (1990). Institutional staff training and management: a review of the literature and a model for geriatric, long-term care facilities. *International Journal of Ageing & Human Development* 30(4) 287-302.

Kitwood T & Woods RT (1995). *A training and development strategy for dementia care in residential settings.* Bradford Dementia Group, Bradford.

Ward T, Murphy E & Procter A (1991). Functional assessment in severely demented patients. *Age & Ageing* 20 212 - 216.

Acknowledgement

This project would not have been possible without the cooperation and participation of staff and residents of the Bradbury Centre, Shepperton, and of RSAS AgeCare, who sponsored the project. We are most grateful to them all.

• Published in *JDC*, March/April 2000.

27 An evaluation of the ExtraCare activity challenge

DAWN BROOKER

ExtraCare Charitable Trust, which provides a variety of care options for older people in the UK, has many years' experience of taking elderly residents with physical disabilities on activity holidays, where the emphasis is on challenge and achievement.

HOW DCM WAS USED
TO EVALUATE A SCHEME
WHICH TOOK PEOPLE
WITH DEMENTIA FOR AN
OUTDOOR ACTIVITY
HOLIDAY

ExtraCare has developed a good relationship with a centre called the Calvert Trust in Devon and uses it for challenge experiences and as a holiday centre throughout the year. The staff at ExtraCare view these experiences very positively for elderly residents who are physically frail. They report that residents gain enormous increases in self-esteem from their achievements at Calvert.

Over the past few years ExtraCare has been particularly keen to develop the best ways of providing fulfilling lives for its residents with dementia. As an organisation, it has made an investment in training and developing staff skills in person-centred care. ExtraCare staff were keen to know whether the kind of improvements in self-esteem and well-being their physically frail residents had shown could be gained by residents with dementia participating in the Calvert experience .

The practice of person-centred care has come a long way in the last 10 years. Activity and occupation are now seen as central to promoting well-being for people with dementia. Care practitioners spend much time in discussing what is the best type of occupation to provide. Going on holiday, however, with all of the rich experiences that this activity can provide, has not been systematically evaluated as an experience for people with dementia.

There is a conventional wisdom in dementia care that familiar routines and environments are important in the maintenance of well-being. This argument can be put forward for not organising holidays at all. Alternatively, holidays are organised which amount to little more than putting people on a coach and transferring them to have the same experiences as they have in their residential care in another location. Activity holidays, with an emphasis on outdoor pursuits and challenge, may have been in vogue for team-building management teams but they are not usually on the agenda for people with dementia.

The activity centre

The Calvert Trust is fully adapted for wheelchair users. It has communal dining and sitting areas with a clubroom and a bar. Sleeping accommodation is in adapted en suite bedrooms that overlook a safe central courtyard area. The experience at Calvert Trust is not a gentle pursuit of day trips and snoozing in the sun. Daytime activities consist of canoeing, hot air ballooning, pony trap riding, abseiling, the zip wire, swimming in the heated pool and the jacuzzi. Trips are organised to a local working farm to feed the animals, and to the seaside with walks up and down the prom. The staff are experienced in providing a safe environment in which people with disabilities can participate in these activities. On the five-day break that is described here, residents were encouraged to take part in at least two activities a day and were organised into small teams with each team following the same programme of activities at different times. Each evening there was a programme of professional entertainment and the bar was open.

Evaluating the impact of care practices on people with dementia is particularly difficult. Because of the problems with language and memory that are part of dementia, people with moderate or severe dementia cannot necessarily say verbally if they find a particular activity satisfying or aversive. In order to evaluate the impact of care practice, non-verbal indicators of well-being can be observed. One way in which this can be measured systematically is by using Dementia Care Mapping (DCM) (Bradford Dementia Group 1997). DCM is based on a person-centred philosophy of care (Kitwood 1997). Of the tools that currently exist to help us understand the perspective of the person with dementia living in formal care settings, this one yields the richest picture (Brooker 1995). DCM was used during this evaluation to measure the well-being of residents with dementia before, during and one month after the ExtraCare challenge experience, and to compare their experience with a matched group of residents who remained in the nursing home environment.

The participants

Twenty residents (11 women and nine men) from four different ExtraCare specialist dementia nursing homes were taken on holiday to Calvert Trust in early October

1999. All had a diagnosis of a dementia illness. Six out of the 20 could not give their name on an orientation test, nine could give their name but no other information, the other five could name the town in which they lived also. Half the group was wheelchair dependent or needed significant help in walking. Only two of the group were independent in terms of continence; all the others were very dependent in this area of care. On the survey version of the CAPE (Clifton Assessment Procedures for the Elderly 1979), nine of the participants were in the most dependent category (E), with the remainder scoring in the next highest level of dependency (D). Unfortunately, the plans for one resident had to be changed at the last minute and another resident came in his place. This means there is only comparative before, during and after data for 19 residents.

Staffing and organisation of care

The care was delivered quite differently at Calvert from the nursing homes. Staff from all four homes participated. Staffing ratios were one-to-one throughout the holiday. Mealtimes were social affairs, with staff and residents eating together. The staff also participated in the challenges and the activities during the daytime. During the day, staff and residents wore the same style tracksuits and outdoor wear. At night, there was less care than is usually required within the residents' home setting. The home setting has a minimum staff ratio of one awake staff member to 10 residents at night. At Calvert there were more staff available but they had all worked a full day and were expecting to sleep. Staff and residents also shared their sleeping accommodation. All staff were on call and provided as much care as required.

Measures

DCM (Bradford Dementia Group 1997) was the main measure used during the evaluation. Throughout the study the seventh edition of the DCM method was used as described in Chapter 2. WiB values and scores were used as the main measure in this study.

Many ExtraCare Charitable Trust staff have a qualification in DCM and a further four were trained as part of this project. Mappers achieved a concordance inter-rater reliability of 80 per cent with each other.

Staff impressions of well-being, sleep patterns, continence, mobility, weight, eating pattern, physical health and medication use by residents were also measured before, after and during the holiday.

Design of the evaluation

DCM was used to evaluate the residents' experiences throughout all aspects of the waking day at Calvert. To assess the impact of the holiday the residents were also

Table 1: mean WIB scores before, during and after the Calvert experience

	Before Calvert	During Calvert	One month after
Calvert Group	Mean WIB 1.13	Mean WIB 1.94	Mean WIB 1.19
N=19	Mode 1.4	Mode 1.7 & 2.4	Mode 1 & 1.1
	Range 0.4-1.9	Range 0.5-3.9	Range 0.3-2.7
	SD 0.419	SD 0.795	SD 0.526
Control Group	Mean WIB 1.12		Mean WIB 0.95
N=19	Mode 0.8		Mode 0.9
	Range -0.3-3.4		Range -0.3-2.0
	SD 0.763		SD 0.582

(All figures positive unless minus sign is shown)

Table 2: Statistical analysis – paired t-test results

Test between	Results	Conclusions
Calvert Group t-test before and during Calvert	Paired t-test t=-4.230 df 18 Significant at 0.001 level	WIB scores were significantly higher while the group were at Calvert
Calvert Group t-test during and after Calvert	Paired t-test t=6.127 df 18 Significant at 0.0001 level	WIB scores were significantly higher while the group were at Calvert
Calvert Group t-test before and after Calvert	Paired t-test t=-0.561 df 18 Not significant	There were no significant differences between the WIB scores pre and post Calvert
Control Group t-test before and Calvert	Paired t-test t=1.453 df 17 Not significant	There were no significant differences between the WIB scores pre and post Calvert

mapped for six consecutive hours in the week before their holiday and, for a further six hours, four weeks after they returned. Thus, for each participant, their experience at Calvert could be compared with their usual pattern at home. Any discernible longer-term benefits or increases in ill-being could also be assessed.

To ensure that any changes in the before and after scores would not have occurred simply by chance, a further 20 residents who did not attend the Calvert Trust holiday were also mapped. These residents were mapped at the same points before and after the holiday in the same residential settings as those who went on holiday. In effect, this group of residents was the control group. Also, to ensure that the results were not just picking up staff bias in thinking that those on the holiday had seen lasting benefits, the mappers carrying out the DCM before and after the holiday had no idea which residents had been to Calvert Trust and which had not. These 'blind' mappers were either staff working at different residential establishments who had not been to Calvert or they were mappers bought in specifically as part of this evaluation.

The impact of the holiday

The average Group WIB score ranges and standard deviation for the Calvert and the control group can be found in Table 1. Statistical analysis (Table 2) suggests that, as a group, well-being was significantly higher while participants were at Calvert than beforehand. Out of the 19 par-

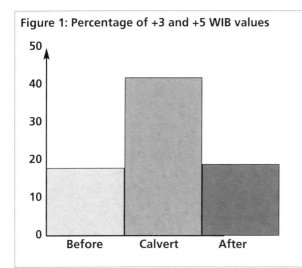

Figure 1: Percentage of +3 and +5 WIB values

Table 3: Relative WIB scores of 19 individuals

WIB score	Before Calvert	During Calvert	One month after
Excellent (≥2.7)	0	11%(2)	5%(1)
Very good (2.1-2.5)	0	37%(7)	0
Good (1.5-2.0)	11%(2)	26%(5)	16%(3)
Fair (0.9-1.4)	63%(12)	21%(4)	58%(11)
Poor (<0.9)	26%(5)	5%(1)	21%(4)

(actual numbers in brackets)

ticipants at Calvert, the well-being scores were improved for 16 of them. Three residents' well-being scores decreased very slightly; these decreases were so slight, however, that they could have been due to chance factors. Eight of the residents achieved significant increases of greater than 1 WIB value overall.

A month after their return from Calvert, residents were mapped in their home environments. All achieved lower scores of well-being than when they were at Calvert Trust but similar scores to those they achieved before the holiday. Statistical analysis (Table 2) suggests that well-being was significantly higher while people were at Calvert compared with a month after.

Of the 18 people in the control group (who did not go to Calvert but were mapped at the same points in time), 10 of their well-being scores decreased over time, three stayed exactly the same and five increased. Most changes were slight.

The average WIB scores for the two groups before and after Calvert can be found in Table 1. Statistical analysis

---

Figure 2: Observations by staff of participants at Calvert Trust

- Staff rated all residents' general well-being as improved
- 3 significantly improved sleep
- 3 significantly improved continence
- 3 significantly improved mobility
- 8 ate better
- 5 gained weight and 2 lost it

Figure 3: 'What happened to people' – some examples

- At home, Hugo is usually pushed around in his wheel-chair. He spent most of his time during the Activity Challenge on his feet. In the evening he took to the dance floor, as he did when he used to be a competitive dancer.
- Maggie, a very frail lady, went down the zip wire and wanted more. She went down a second time. That evening, she sang her heart out with the entertainment - reliving memories of amateur operatics
- Bert – after a trip in the hot air balloon – did five lengths of the pool, shunned the steps, athletically pushing himself out the pool. Later, in the bar, he started speaking fluent Italian – a talent no one knew he had.

---

suggests that well-being was significantly higher while people were at Calvert compared with levels both before and after the experience. Their well-being did not significantly change as a result of the Calvert experience in the long-term.

In terms of the quality of experiences for individuals, a rough guide is provided within the DCM method for what these scores equate to. More individuals could be seen to be having a more positive experience at Calvert than at home. The numbers of WIB scores falling within the respective categories are shown in Table 3.

The percentage of WIB values falling within +3 and +5 categories (indicating positive signs of well-being as opposed to absence of ill-being) was much higher at Calvert as demonstrated in Figure 1.

The staff views

The staff were all of the opinion that their residents benefited from their experiences on holiday. Staff reported that three out of the 19 had significant improvements in sleep, continence and mobility. The others' patterns remained unchanged although one person experienced slightly decreased mobility while on holiday. Eight people ate better on holiday and this was maintained for at least two people on their return home. Five people put weight on over the holiday and two lost a little. There was little change in people's general health or medication intake. These are summarised in Figure 2.

The practical experiences of staff revealed that the residents slept significantly better and required far less care during the night time than they would have at home. It is certainly the case that the entire relationship of care changed at Calvert Trust.

What happened to some individuals

There were some remarkable stories of improved well-being at Calvert Trust which cannot be expressed in terms of quantitative data. Figure 3 details some of these.

Some residents' levels of well-being increased dramatically while they were on holiday. From the data available there did not seem to be a particular factor which predicted who would enjoy the holiday the most. These 'super holidaymakers' were a mixed group in terms of gender, the homes they came from and their level of disability and dementia. It may be that a more detailed scrutiny of their histories would reveal some common themes.

What made a difference at Calvert?

It is unlikely that this sort of holiday would have been experienced by many of the residents prior to the onset of their dementia. There may well have been aspects, however, that brought back very positive earlier memories. For example, being around horses and animals and being on the water may well have been a feature of childhood holidays for many. Certainly the ease with which many residents swam was a joy to watch. Watching the excitement on the face of one elderly lady being fixed into her harness on the zip wire by an attractive male instructor was more difficult to explain by reference to earlier memory. However, the exhilaration of travelling fast with the wind in your face probably beats any sensory experience that can be achieved in a multi-sensory room. Sitting in a bar with a pint of beer looked a very familiar activity for many.

The Calvert experience was unique in many respects. The staff:resident ratio at Calvert was much higher than in the usual residential setting and the whole day was spent with residents in activity. In fact, there was a feeling that the staff and the resident group were living together for this period. Staff were challenged by the Calvert experience too. Feedback from staff is that everyone feels 'an equal' at Calvert Trust and the traditional relationship of 'carer' and 'passive recipient' disappears. There was a feeling that everyone, regardless of disability, was in this together.

Longer-term changes

By and large there was no significant lasting impact on well-being over time as measured by DCM. Perhaps, given the dependence on present environment in determining well-being for people with dementia, this is not surprising. Residents with physical frailty but no memory impairment have the opportunity to relive the experience through talking about their achievements with family and friends. This is not an option for residents with the degree of dementia suffered by those who took part in this evaluation.

For some staff, the positive experiences of seeing the potential for well-being in certain residents for the first time will have had longer lasting effects in the way in which staff and residents relate to each other. Unfortunately, DCM could not have monitored this sort of subtle change in practice. This is not to say that there would not have been lasting benefits. The likelihood is that these benefits would accrue over time. It could also be expected that because the visit to Calvert Trust was such an extraordinary experience in the lives of both staff and residents who participated, it will live on in the emotional memories of both groups. It will be interesting to see how residents react when they return to Calvert Trust. It may well be that it will be an even more positive experience for them the second time around.

A long-term aim would be to replicate the increase in well-being experienced by the residents who went to Calvert Trust in their home setting. Although it would not be possible to recreate the Calvert experience in its entirety, there are elements that could be repeated more frequently at home. An investigation of the care maps could identify particular episodes of well-being. It could be investigated whether an activity co-ordinator could use residents' experiences at Calvert Trust to provide them with activities which elevate their well-being in the ways it was raised on holiday.

Staff returning from Calvert Trust can reflect on residents' experiences and write care plans which explicitly detail the activities which enhanced residents' well-being. It may also be that making home-based activities feature the outdoors and include more physical elements may have an equally beneficial effect. Continued use of Dementia Care Mapping would provide evidence about whether these goals can be achieved.

A further investigation of why some residents benefited to such a great extent could also be illuminating in selecting further residents for the ExtraCare activity challenge.

Conclusions

This evaluation has shown beyond doubt that the Calvert Trust holiday was a very valuable experience for those residents who participated. This bears out the subjective experience of the staff and the evaluators seeing the great enjoyment and social time that people had. The vast majority of participants had a great time, with a significant proportion demonstrating a potential for well-being that no one had previously seen. There were no participants whose well-being was significantly decreased by the holiday experience either in the short or longer term.

Staff evaluation of improvements in physical well-being confirm the view that this was a positive experience. This can be set in contrast to the effects on well-being that periods of 'respite care' often have on people with dementia. The positive impact on psychological and physical functioning seen at Calvert is not the norm when people with dementia are taken out of familiar environments. Something very positive happened to ExtraCare residents at Calvert.

• Adapted from an article published in *JDC*, May/June 2001.

References

Bradford Dementia Group (1997) *Evaluating Dementia Care: The DCM Method*. Seventh Edition. University of Bradford.

Brooker DJR (1995) Looking at them, looking at me: A review of observational studies into the quality of institutional care for elderly people with dementia. *Journal of Mental Health* 4 145-156.

Kitwood T (1997) *Dementia Reconsidered*. Open University Press, Buckingham.

Kitwood T, Bredin K (1992) A new approach to the evaluation of dementia care. *Journal of Advances in Health and Nursing Care* 1 41-60.

Pattie AH & Gilleard CJ (1979) *Manual of the Clifton Assessment Procedures for the Elderly (CAPE)*. Hodder and Stoughton, Sevenoaks.

28 Sensory stimulation groups: do the benefits last?

SIOBHAIN MAGUIRE, ANNA-LOUISE GOSLING

Increasing levels of well-being for people in the later stages of dementia, by providing activity and stimulation, can be a difficult task and some may argue a pointless one. This article reports on an activity and stimulation group set up in a nursing home for a small group of residents.

In the previous decade, the benefits of activity and stimulation on quality of life for people with dementia have been well recognised. However, many care settings lack purposeful activity (Brooker 1995) and staff may not be aware of its role in maintaining quality of life. When activity programmes take place, people in the later stages of dementia are sometimes excluded or involved inappropriately. Questions are often asked such as: 'Why does such a client group need a programme of activities anyway? What would be the point?' (Challis 1996). When activity programmes are introduced their role and potential benefits are often unknown. It is therefore important to evaluate and disseminate methods used to improve well-being and quality of life in people with dementia.

Morgan and Stewart (1997) have identified the need for appropriate levels of activity and stimulation as necessary components in maintaining a good quality of life. Further, they reported a carry-over effect that well-being lasts after such activities.

However the correlation between activity and quality of life is not so simple. Brooker (1995) argues that participation in inappropriate activities cannot enhance quality of life. Simply looking at people's activity levels is not sufficient to infer their level of well-being.

Measuring well-being and quality of life for people in the later stages of dementia poses both conceptual and methodological difficulties (Green 1995; Selai & Trimble 1999). For instance, language is often severely impaired (Copeland et al 1990; Goldsmith 1996), so interviews and questionnaires present problems. Direct observation of behaviour (Perrin 1997) may help but what behaviours indicate increased levels of well-being? How do you account for individual differences of expression? The structured observational technique of DCM helps overcome some of these difficulties. It has not, however, been fully explored to work with people in the later stages of dementia (Bradford Dementia Group 1997).

> DO THE BENEFITS OF RUNNING AN ACTIVITY AND STIMULATION GROUP HAVE ANY DEMONSTRABLE EFFECT AFTER THE GROUP HAS FINISHED?

Aims of study

We set up an activity and stimulation group for people in the later stages of dementia, to see if they could be engaged and if their levels of well-being could be maintained after the group had finished.

The nursing home where this study took place has 72 residents (60 people with dementia and 12 with severe and enduring mental health problems). Residents have a variety of physical and psychological needs, including the presentation of 'challenging behaviour'. The nursing home is divided into six different units, each providing accommodation for 12 residents.

The group

The activity group was intended to have a minimum of four, and a maximum of six residents attend each week. Members' average age was 83, with an age range of 61 to 92. Residents' backgrounds were researched and recorded into an activity file. This helped structure the group and tailor activities according to interest and need. Residents' activity plans were reviewed and updated regularly as the group progressed and more information was obtained. Members had fluctuating levels of mood, perception, communication, motivation and physical needs.

All the residents in the study had a diagnosis of a dementia (one of whom had early onset dementia). In an attempt to categorise their level of impairment (for this study), Pool's Activity Level Instrument (PAL) was used (Pool 1999). Completion of the PAL checklist establishes where the person with dementia is operating at one of four activity levels; planned, exploratory, sensory and reflex. The group's members were functioning at the sensory level. Briefly, this suggests that the person may not have many thoughts or ideas about carrying out an activity, but will be mainly concerned with experiencing sensations. Under close direction, he or she can possibly carry out single-step tasks (Pool 1999).

The group was run in one of the units that was said to receive the least activity input due to the overall level of deterioration of the residents. All its residents were women. The groups ran at a regular time and place every week. The structure was that four to six residents would be asked to go from the lounge into the 'quiet room' where an

Themes for the group activities
- Hats and personal care – looking at and trying on a variety of hats and scarves, make-up and jewellery.
- Holidays – including tactile materials related to holiday theme, old postcards and photographs, relevant music
- Fashion – including fashion magazines, mannequin templates, material samples
- Tea/coffee group - with objects reminiscent of past tea times, music and old magazines, eg Picture Post
- Music – involving various musical instruments and different types of music
- Touch and smell – including perfumes, aromatherapy oils, herbs and spices, various textured materials and objects.

activity would be set up. The group ran for approximately 30 to 45 minutes, depending on levels of engagement. Due to the group's social and stimulation format, it came to be called 'the social and sensory stimulation group'.

The group met some initial reluctance from residents and staff. It took approximately three months for the group to develop a routine and structure that the residents (and staff) seemed to enjoy. Once the group had become established, some residents started to show signs of awareness about the group. Comments were made to the facilitators such as 'are all us girls going there again?'. Other residents showed increased awareness by their facial expressions or actions. It appeared that the group was successful in achieving its aims and additionally was having an impact on residents whose level of deterioration was previously thought to be too impaired to benefit from group interactions. It is for this reason that the group was more formally evaluated.

Results

Group members were observed in the lounge for 30 minutes before the group started and for 30 minutes in the lounge after the group had finished. People were not observed when moving from the lounge to the group room nor if they left either the group room or the lounge.

Data from all six observation sessions have been aggregated into three categories: before the group, during the group and after the group.

Table 1 shows the number of time frames spent in the five most frequent behaviour categories for before, during and after the group, it also expresses these as a percentage.

Before and after the group the percentage of time spent in the top five categories is lower, indicating a broader range of activities.

Although residents were engaged in a wider range of activities during these times, the top five categories show that they were less meaningful than those during the group. For example, some of the top five categories before and after the group included sleeping or dozing, being socially involved but passively and repetitive self-stimulation. This compares with direct engagement of the senses and engaging in expressive or creative activity, which were major activities during the group.

The category 'interacting verbally or otherwise' features in all three conditions and may be misleading. More time was spent in this category before the group (15.4 per cent) than during (11.1 per cent) or after (11.4 per cent). This tells us little about the quality of interaction or level of engagement. For instance, the category interacting verbally or otherwise is scored regardless of whether the whole five minutes is spent engaged in meaningful interaction, or social contact is simply a brief 'hello'. Looking at the well- and ill-being values helps to clarify this apparent discrepancy.

Well- and ill-being values can help define quality of interaction and engagement. They are recorded on a six-point scale. These values can be converted to well- and ill-being (WIB) scores, which are an average for any given time period.

Residents' well-being scores were higher during the group than before or after. Once the group had finished, scores dropped to similar levels before the group.

For example, Mrs M had well-being scores of 0.84 before the group, 2.42 during the group and a score of 1 afterwards. Residents spent most of their time in WIB value 3

Table 1: Top 5 behaviour categories before, during and after the group		
Behaviour category code	No of 5-minute time frames spent in category	Time spent in category as a percentage
BEFORE THE GROUP		
Receiving practical, physical or personal care	27	16.7%
Interacting verbally or otherwise – with no other obvious activity	25	15.4%
Being socially involved, but passively	20	12.3%
Repetitive self stimulation	18	11.1%
Engaging with media	17	10.5%
DURING THE GROUP		
Direct engagement of the senses	51	25.8%
Engaging with media	39	19.7%
Engaging in expressive or creative activity	37	18.7%
Receiving practical, physical or personal care	33	16.7%
Interacting verbally or otherwise – with no other obvious activity	22	11.1%
AFTER THE GROUP		
Engaging with media	19	14.4%
Sleeping, dozing	18	13.6%
Interacting verbally or otherwise – with no other obvious activity	15	11.4%
	14	10.6%
Receiving practical, physical or personal care	14	10.6%

during the group, while they spent the majority of their time in WIB value 1 before and after the group. This suggests the group had a positive effect on well-being while it was happening.

Discussion

Not surprisingly this study shows that residents spent more time engaged during the group than before or after it. This is reflected by significant increases in levels of well-being. People in the later stages of dementia thus can benefit from activity and stimulation if provided in an appropriate way. This links in with Kitwood's (1997) person-centred care approach, that people in the later stages of dementia need increased levels of support, specifically aimed at meeting psychological needs.

These results contribute to others' findings (eg Brooker et al 1998) that appropriate activity and stimulation lead to improved levels of well-being and thus quality of life.

However, levels of well-being achieved during the group were not maintained in the immediate period of time after the group, thus no carry-over effect was found. This could be explained in a number of ways. Firstly, some of the members were reluctant, when the group ended, to leave the room. Secondly, practice altered slightly throughout the study – previously when the group ended and residents returned to the lounge the facilitators spent some time in the area 'winding down'. During the study the facilitators did not spend any time after the group in the lounge to enable post group measures to be taken.

Thirdly, the end of the group coincided with toileting. Often, as residents were escorted back to the lounge, staff took the opportunity to take them to the toilet. This resulted in many residents looking anxious and becoming restless.

Finally, it could be that there was no carry-over effect. Perhaps looking for a carry-over effect removes the value of the 'here and now' experience. For people with dementia, the future often does not hold much appeal, either due to an inability to plan ahead, or to remember much of the past, so the here and now takes on more significance. Perhaps the aim, when working with people in the later stages of dementia, should be to increase 'here and now' moments. This has implications for staff training, in that it highlights the need for a care environment that offers opportunities for interaction and stimulation throughout the day.

Although this study used Dementia Care Mapping (DCM) as its method of evaluation, its use has not been fully explored with people in the later stages of dementia (Bradford Dementia Group 1997). By using DCM dramatic increases in well-being were observed. However, some subtle changes in behaviour were not recorded. This is because DCM is not designed to record minor differences in behaviour, which are more often seen in the later stages of dementia. This further highlights the conceptual and methodological difficulties when working with people in this stage. Perrin (1997) has suggested a possible alternative that may be more appropriate when evaluating quality of life in the later stages of dementia: 'the positive response schedule for severe dementia'.

In conclusion, the social and sensory stimulation group achieved its aim to improve quality of life by increasing well-being. It re-emphasised the importance of providing activity and stimulation and the value of working within the here and now.

• Published in *JDC*, March/April 2003.

Acknowledgements

We should like to thank all the residents who took part in the study, Stephanie Hall, occupational therapist, for her invaluable ideas and help, Dr Martin Skelton-Robinson and Catherine Somerville for their thoughts and general help and acknowledge the valuable feedback received at the PSIGE conference.

References

Bradford Dementia Group (1997) *Dementia Care Mapping Manual*, 7th Edition. University of Bradford.

Brooker D, Foster N, Banner A, Payne M, Jackson L. (1998) The efficacy of dementia care mapping as an audit tool: report of a 3 year British NHS evaluation. *Aging and Mental Health* 2 (1) 60-70.

Brooker D (1995) Looking at them, looking at me. A review of observational studies in to the quality of institutional care for elderly people with dementia. *Journal of Mental Health* 4 145-156.

Challis T (1996) Purposeful activity and elderly mentally ill people: why? *British Journal of Occupational Therapy* 59(4) 183-184.

Copeland JRM, Crosby C, Sixmith AJ (1990) *Three experimental homes for the elderly mentally ill: final report*. Institute of Human Ageing, Liverpool.

Goldsmith M (1996) *Hearing the voice of people with dementia*. Jessica Kingsley, London.

Green S (1995) Elderly mentally ill people and quality of life: who wants activities? *British Journal of Occupational Therapy* 58 (9) 377-382.

Kitwood T (1997) *Dementia reconsidered*. Open University Press, Buckingham.

Morgan DG, Stewart NJ (1997) The importance of the social environment in dementia care. *Western Journal of Nursing Research* 19 (6) 740-761.

Perrin T (1997) The positive response schedule for severe dementia. *Aging and Mental Health* 1(2) 184-191.

Pool J (1999) *A user guide to the Pool's Activity Levels (PAL) Checklist and Action Plan for people with dementia*. Bradford Dementia Group Good Practice Guides.

Selai C and Trimble MR (1999) Assessing quality of life in dementia. *Aging and Mental Health* 3(2) 101-111.

29 Lifted into a world of rhythm and melody

TESSA PERRIN

I sat watching a Jabadao dance and movement session run by Sandy Crichton (see box opposite), wondering what on earth Sandy could do with such a large, disparate group of people. There was a distinct air of grumpiness in the ward atmosphere that afternoon. Ivy was particularly irritable, holding forth in a non-stop diatribe against the world in general and anybody who happened to cross her line of vision in particular.

THE AUTHOR RECORDED AND ANALYSED HER OBSERVATIONS OF A JABADAO DANCE AND MOVEMENT SESSION

Lily had argued with someone over lunch, and taken herself off in a huff to sit alone at the farthest end of the corridor. Extracted from her chair with great difficulty, she now joined the gathering group reluctantly, eyeing people suspiciously as she took her place in the circle. She fell under Ivy's gaze and was subjected to a torrent of abuse, but was quite able to return the compliment, and a loud and vitriolic argument began to gather momentum. Other patients in the group were starting to look anxious or bewildered, or to become similarly belligerent, according to their ability to relate to what was going on. A few others were withdrawn; if they were conscious of the disturbance, there was no sign.

In the middle of all this, Sandy was attempting to greet and exchange pleasantries with each new patient to arrive. I felt anxious for her, and uncomfortable for myelf. I knew that if this Jabadao session had been my responsibility, I would be wishing myself miles away at this moment. I had been working alongside Sandy for several weeks, conducting formal observations of the Jabadao approach (Crichton 1997) as she worked with twos and threes of the more severely impaired patients on the ward. This was the first large group session where the invitation was open. It had actually grown much larger than originally intended, but Sandy appeared unfazed by the gathering.

With everyone gathered and introductions over, Sandy put some music on, some rather bouncy, foot-tappy accordion music that reminded me of English country dancing lessons of childhood. Immediately, the palpable tension broke and spirits seemed to lift. Ivy and Lily quit griping and haranguing each other and began to respond to the music. It was as though somebody had thrown a switch, which I suppose in a sense they had. I was astonished.

At first Sandy moved around the circle, using some of the gentle one-to-one techniques I had observed in the small group work, picking up people's responses, echoing and reflecting, encouraging and stretching each individual's chosen movements in verbal, visual and (where permitted) physical contact. Then Lily got up, picked up her skirts, and, whooping in true country-dance fashion, started to dance and kick her legs in the air. Ivy did the same; suddenly, and curiously, they were the best of friends.

Sandy was quick to pick up the cue, and leaped into the dance herself. Out came the floaty rainbow scarves (one for everyone) which were waved and thrown, twisted and wrapped, knotted and looped as each chose to use them; then in turn came the twizzle sticks, the balloons and finally the parachute. Fifteen or twenty minutes into the session, most people were participating and there was a joyful air of what can perhaps best be described as festivity.

Frank, unsmiling as usual, was nevertheless grabbing eagerly for the equipment, and totally taken up with the parachute when it appeared. Flo, who rarely does anything except sit in a heap, or perhaps wail and scream, smiled benignly throughout, waving her twizzle stick in time to the music. Alice, frosty at first, at last unfolded her arms from her chest and started to experiment with the different shapes and textures moving about her. When the balloon came her way, she sent it back with some energy. Iris, not quite so free, was unable to open up in the same physical way, but was clearly locked into the music, smiling and swaying in her chair, from time to time breaking into a beautiful rich alto. Her song didn't always match the music, but it didn't matter; she was lost in a world of rhythm and melody.

Not everyone enjoyed the Jabadao experience. Arthur had only arrived for a respite stay an hour or two earlier, and looked distinctly uncomfortable throughout. For him, it was probably a chaotic and disorientating exercise which must have been unhelpful. But he was the only group member for whom it appeared to be a negative experience. There were two or three other, severely impaired people whom the experience passed by, as we might have expected, eliciting neither positive nor negative response.

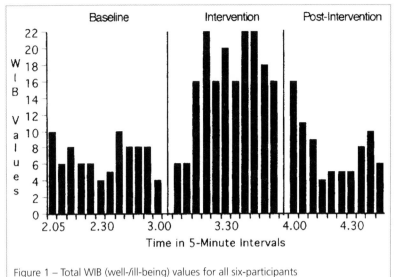

Figure 1 – Total WIB (well-/ill-being) values for all six-participants

converts data into individual and group scores, or into a profile which examines the distribution of WIB values across the continuum of +5 +3 +1 -1 -3 -5. Neither of these methods would enable us to look at the impact on the general well-being of the group across the intervention, so I chose to total the WIB values for all six participants in each individual time frame, and present the data as a bar chart (Fig 1).

One naturally returns to the raw data sheets to examine the impact on each individual, but it is clear from the above that for the group generally there was a significant improvement in well-being for the duration of the session. The raw data also show that for three participants there was a rich spread of "that +5 feeling" (Barnett 1995) intermingled with +3s. Only one client was unable to rise above a +1, and there were no negative values during the period of intervention.

Before the large group session, I had been observing Sandy's work with some of the most severely impaired patients on the ward. This was in the context of a research project designed to measure the impact of different occupations on well-being in severe dementia. For recording these observations I used the Positive Response Schedule for Severe Dementia (Perrin 1997) a tool designed specifically for monitoring the well-being of severely impaired people.

The Positive Response Schedule picks up the component parts of complex behaviours; that is, it won't distinguish between feeding or dressing or listening to music, as dementia care mapping does, but it will record the physical, emotional and interactive behaviours elicited during

But for the greater number, it had been a dynamic and joyful interlude.

Within five minutes of the session finishing, Ivy and Lily were back at each other's throats, all peace and harmony of relationship destroyed. Had I not actually seen it, I could not have guessed that they had just held hands and laughed and danced together.

Impact on well-being

I had been using Dementia Care Mapping (DCM) (Kitwood and Bredin 1992) to monitor six of the participants within the large group, three of whom would be described as moderately impaired, and three as severely impaired, according to the CAPE Behaviour Rating Scale. The conventional processing of "WIB" values in DCM (scores assigned to a behaviour indicating the relative level of well- or ill- being)

What is JABADAO?

We are a company that has pioneered movement-based work with elderly people in residential and day care settings. We have been dancing, for want of a better word, for more than a decade, with elderly people with dementia.

I believe that the JABADAO approach has a unique contribution to make in enhancing relationships for both clients with dementia and their care staff. The core belief underlying this approach is that dance offers a fundamental yet direct and ordinary means to communicate with each other; an age-old, ageless language common to us all.

I am not talking ballet here. By dance I mean the everyday, continuous, spontaneous movement and body language by which we all express ourselves all the time.

We work with very young people and people with learning disabilities as well as with elderly people and those with dementia; all groups where verbal language is lost, difficult or undeveloped. Movement language may be their only means to express directly who they are and how they are. We believe that non-verbal movement language is a medium we all use all the time and mostly ignore. At JABADAO the spotlight is on movement conversation.

In dementia care settings I am aiming to establish, maintain and develop reationships. Moving is the language I use; communication is my goal.

What does the JABADAO approach offer someone with dementia?

It offers a means of rich communication without the necessity of speech; an avenue of direct communication through movement. When words no longer flow easily, or become unreliable and treacherous, this is painful for all concerned. Using movement to communicate can be a relief and a release ...

When I go into institutional settings, I see people eager for contact... Verbal dialogue may not be possible. Moving talk is. When I work, I am aiming to make contact, move with and be moved by clients. I am starting from where they are, not from how I would like them to be. I am looking for the movement they are offering, not imposing my agenda.

From 'Moving is the language I use – communication is my goal' by Sandy Crichton, project worker and trainer for JABADAO. *Journal of Dementia Care* (November/December 1997) 5(6) 16-17.

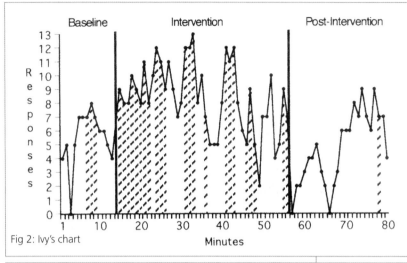

Fig 2: Ivy's chart

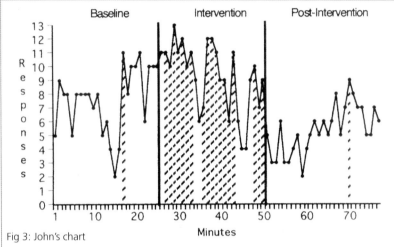

Fig 3: John's chart

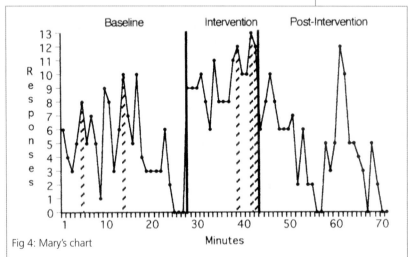

Fig 4: Mary's chart

tive and humour. Please note that the shaded areas on the charts indicate "happy".

For John and for Iris also it was a very positive intervention, but quite different in character. There was the same intensity of response, but manifested in a less flamboyant, more restrained fashion. Iris was able to engage deeply with the music, which at times brought tears to her eyes. John (Fig 3) was less able to engage with the music, but more able to sustain prolonged interaction with Sandy. For Iris it was the music that satisfied; for John, the personal contact.

For Mary and for Frank too, this experience held some pleasure and purpose, though clearly to a lesser extent than for the others; Mary and Frank are both significantly impaired. Neither patient seemed to notice the music, but their pockets of pleasure and increased enjoyment were in each case related to the one-to-one personal interactions with Sandy. Mary's chart is shown in Fig 4.

Observations were conducted with four other very severely impaired patients who might be described as in, or approaching, a vegetative state. Findings from these observations were equivocal and very difficult to interpret. It would appear that the experience had very little effect, positive or negative, on any of them. This was unsurprising; the greater the impairment, the more diminished the response.

The Jabadao approach has much to commend it. It is in a very real sense a person-centred and person-led approach in which agency and control are firmly in the participants' hands. Its emphasis on non-verbal communication renders it accessible to all but the most severe levels of impairment in dementia. It is possible, of course, that it is of value even at these levels. We simply don't have

feeding or dressing or listening to music. It is a tool that may be used fairly reliably over short periods of time (one to two hours) to monitor the impact of specific interventions.

Twelve people were observed in all; in each case across an initial baseline period, the intervention period, and a post-intervention period. For Lily and Ivy, the two more able patients mentioned above, it was a highly positive experience (Ivy's chart is shown in Fig 2). In both cases, there were laughter and smiles, dancing and singing, initia-

measures of sufficient sensitivity to tackle the inward world of the very damaged person. Jabadao is a vibrant experience, dynamic and elemental, colourful and tactile; it is about letting go, it is about being, being yourself just as you are, and being valued, just as you are.

Jabadao is all these things; but I have wondered if its secret is more in person than technique, in the activity leader more than the activity. For above all things I have been impressed with the exquisite courtesy of the approach, the equality of attention to all participants no matter how damaged or overtly objectionable, the self-confident use of body and voice, the skilled reading of atmosphere and ambience, the agility and flexibility of response. We may learn the techniques and exercises without undue difficulty; but we must surely look within for the wherewithal to instill life into the mechanics.

Increasingly in my work as an occupational therapist, I perceive the occupation as subordinate to the personal interaction; this is not to devalue occupation, but to understand the pre-eminent worth of the personal contact within the occupation. This is a client group which, by and large, is dependent upon others for their participation and engagement and well-being in occupations. It is not a group which will solicit or make its own; it requires us to be the channel.

Our motivation therefore, our enthusiasm, our confidence, our inter-personal skills, are the critical factors for engaging dementing people in positive occupations. Jabadao has much to offer the person with dementia. It has much to offer the carer. It is above all a reflective and reciprocal approach; if we can let it teach and release and liberate us, as we hope that it will liberate our clients, we will surely have discovered a truly creative communion.

• Published in JDC, *Jan/Feb* 1998.

References

Barnett E (1995) A window of insight into quality care. *Journal of Dementia Care* 3(4) 23-26.

Kitwood T, Bredin K (1992) A new approach to dementia care. *Journal of Advances in Health and Nursing Care* 1(5) 41-60.

Perrin T (1997) The Positive Response Schedule for Severe Dementia. *Aging and Mental Health* 1(2) 184-191.

Crichton, S (1997) Moving is the language I use – communication is my goal. *Journal of Dementia Care* 5(6) 16-17.

30 Maps from around the world

IDENTIFYING STRENGTHS AND WEAKNESSES

AUSTRALIA

AILEEN WRIGHT shows how she has used DCM to evaluate a diversional therapy programme in a residential care facility in Tasmania. Here the DCM data is used as an outcome measure of practice.

This map took place at Sandown Apartments, a 60 bed high/low care residential facility **1**. The results of the map are extremely beneficial to the Diversional Therapy Programme **2** as they identify the strengths and the weaknesses of the programme.

Some residents may not be gaining maximum benefit because they may be on the fringe of the group, unable to initiate social interaction or participate in activities without continual prompting and encouragement. The map will identify passive participation and unacceptable states of being and the need for the introduction of different strategies to obtain optimum results.

The mapping promotes knowledge of how the resident is actually feeling, what they are experiencing during a particular time, and in harmony with the person-centred approach each person is seen as a unique individual with special skills, interests and needs. The map also gives insights into what is enjoyable for each person or what may trigger a particular behaviour pattern and the variance of well/ill-being at certain times of the day, eg. morning/afternoon or late afternoon/early evening.

The map portrays a clear picture of how the quality of life and the care of residents can be improved and what is needed to bring about changes in the well-being of residents. Certain behaviour category codes recurring over a six hour period can indicate that there is very little happening for residents, and even though activities are provided, these may not be well-organised, sustained or available to everyone.

My best experience using DCM has been with a small group of residents, where a DCM evaluation was undertaken for the second time in three months and recorded a vast increase in state of well-being and interactive behaviour category codes (A, E, G, H, I, J). There were only five residents in the group at this time (4-6pm) and mapping was conducted over three days with each resident recording positive scores for the whole period. During the first evaluation (three months prior) fewer positives were recorded and considerable periods of time elapsed with very little happening.

My worst experience occurred recently when I conducted a DCM evaluation between 12 noon and 6pm with residents with diverse care needs. During the first four hours there was practically nothing happening, staff were few and far between and residents were left solely to their own devices which constituted meal time, reading, little social interaction and sleeping/dozing. I found this experience disturbing and frustrating but I was extremely pleased to have access to a tool which clearly portrayed the situation and demonstrated the need for team discussion to improve the quality of life for the residents.

Most personal detractors I have observed have been in the mild to medium categories and usually relate to:

Disempowerment, Infantilisation, Outpacing, Ignoring

All the majority of personal detractors are inflicted unintentionally without any intent of malice.

I am absolutely thrilled with the DCM process and as I am gaining confidence and mapping more, I feel the sky will be the limit for what can be achieved.

1 mixed nursing home and residential facility; **2** programme provided by a qualified therapist who provides activities for people with disabilities.

Date: 11.6.02 Time Period: 4.00 – 6.00 pm Place: Sandy Glen No. Participants: 26 No. Staff: 4 Observer: Aileen Wright

Participant Name	Time	4.00	4.05	4.10	4.15	4.20	4.25	4.30	4.35	4.40	4.45	4.50	4.55	5.00	5.05	5.10	5.15	5.20	5.25	5.30	5.35	5.40	5.45	5.50	5.55	ΣWIB / ΣTF
Dora	BCC	F	F	G	G	G	G	G	G	G	G	X	X	F	F	F	F	F	F	V	V	V	B	B	B	
	WIB	+1	+1	+3	+3	+3	+3	+3	+3	+3	+3	+3	+3	+3	+3	+3	+3	+3	+3				+3	+3	+3	
Florence	BCC	F	F	G	G	G	G	G	G	G	G	X	X	F	F	F	F	F	F	L	L	L	L	M	M	
	WIB	+1	+1	+3	+3	+3	+3	+3	+3	+3	+3	+3	+3	+3	+3	+3	+3	+3	+3	+3	+3	+3	+3	+1	+1	
Beverley	BCC	F	F	G	G	G	G	G	B	B	B	P	P	F	F	F	F	F	F	L	L	L	L	M	M	
	WIB	+1	+1	+3	+3	+3	+3	+5	+3	+3	+3	+3	+3	+3	+3	+3	+3	+3	+3	+3	+3	+3	+3	+1	+1	
Margaret	BCC	F	F	G	G	G	G	G	B	B	B	P	P	F	F	F	F	F	F	M	M	M	M	M	M	
	WIB	+1	+1	+1	+1	+3	+3	+3	+3	+3	+3	+3	+3	+3	+3	+3	+3	+3	+3	+1	+1	+1	+3	+3	+3	
Evelyn	BCC	F	F	G	G	G	G	G	G	G	G	K	K	F	F	F	F	F	F	M	M	M	M	M	M	
	WIB	+1	+1	+1	+1	+1	+1	+1	+1	+1	+1	+1	+1	+3	+3	+3	+3	+3	+3	+1	+1	+3	+3	+3	+3	

Notes

- **PDs** None. Very interactive two hours
- Div Therapist and carer very attentive to the whole group
- Dora active participant in board game – really enjoying
- Evelyn active participant but prompting needed
- Florence really enjoying daily chat after meal.

AN IMPORTANT JOURNEY

ENGLAND

CAROLE DINSHAW describes how she developed DCM within a large mental health trust in England and discusses the process needed to allow DCM to evolve

The ward involved was an 18-bed assessment ward, caring wholly for people with cognitive impairment. It was originally one of many transferred from a large institution five years previously, many of its existing staff transferring with it. It was a bright and airy ward. At the time of the map there were 12 patients and an average of four staff per shift. There was no occupational therapy or clinical psychology input, and staff in the area had had little training. There was a minimal but very supportive physiotherapy input.

I had begun to talk to managers whenever possible about DCM long before the map. Much to my disbelief after seeing it work so successfully elsewhere, there was not a great deal of interest – until my ideas captured the attention of the then lead nurse. The ward manager had been resistant and although I was open and honest about the process and function of DCM, was reluctant to 'let me in' and only seemed reassured by the notion that she was 'helping me with a project'. I moved from her to talk to the other nursing staff, giving verbal and written information. This was not easy and the ward manager did little to help me allay the staff's anxieties at being mapped (that is observed as they saw it). The process was however helped by my doing a shift the day before the map. I made an effort to 'muck in' with everything – that is, did my best to be seen as a 'jobbing' nurse, 'one of them'. At this stage where both the process and I were not known I felt I had made a breakthrough. Not only did I feel less of an outsider; I gained an insight into the environment and the patient group's potential.

I saw some magnificent examples of positive events and some personal detractors that needed immediate attention, which I still refer to anonymously in my training sessions. On a positive note, the skills and approaches of some of the staff were highly encouraging, while those of the ward manager and a doctor concerned me most. The ward manager tried to make a male patient who was being scored as E + 3, listening attentively and humming to music, get up and dance with her. He maintained his wellbeing but only because he argued against this in a very vociferous manner! In another situation, a doctor approached a patient at the table as he was dozing after lunch. Without any communication she lifted his vest up, exposing his bare back to all. She placed a stethoscope on his back. He did not respond and continued to doze, but this fitted perfectly into the 'objectification' personal detractor description. For me, these incidents highlighted the importance of noting everything, however difficult, and not just the interactions that affect the WIB score. Had this been the case these important events would have been lost and not noted for action.

I chose this map for a number of reasons but notably not for its level of perfection or absolute awfulness. I chose it because it gave me an important inroad into using the tool and it was the first where I led the whole process – and the one I probably learned the most from. I also chose it because this ward is now so different. Many of the staff on this ward still work there, though there have been some notable and important changes at a senior level. The last two maps in these areas paint very different pictures. Another reason I chose this map was that it has led one of the staff on to become a basic mapper. Since the map, she has also become an important advocate and active member of the whole process. She has now been promoted and teaches, demonstrates and fosters a person-centred approach to care.

For me, based on what Tom Kitwood had 'started' for me, the map was the beginning of an important journey taking DCM forward in Worcestershire, where it is now an essential part of our quality strategy.

Notes (see charts on next page)

- 0840 VR – 10b. Finger pricked by care staff for blood with no explanation. Spoken to kindly afterwards.
- 0855 WG – 10c. Cream put round mouth with no explanation.
- 0910 BQ – 8a. Porridge put in front, no choice offered. B screwed up her nose and pushed it away.
- 1000 MG – Reassured by care staff and responded "Aren't they fusspots!"
- 1010 BQ – Asked observer questions re other patients.
- 1005 WG – Breakfast taken away. Care staff: "will be lunch before he finishes!" 7b
- 1105 Staff started playing dominoes and word game. BQ and MG encouraged in activity through to 1145.
- 1045 EJ – 15a Forced to get up and dance.
- 1205 WG – 12c Pushed to sit down.
- 1245 WG – 2c Pushed food in.
- 1255 WG – 2c Dinner taken away despite him still eating.
- 1320 VC – 10d Examined by dr at table. No explanation.
- 1335 EJ – 8a Music turned down. E momentarily cross.

Date: 1.10.98 Time Period: 0755-0955 Place: No. Participants: 12 No. Staff: 3 + 1 agency Observer: Carole

Participant Name	Time	0800	0805	0810	0815	0820	0825	0830	0835	0840	0845	0850	0855	0900	0905	0910	0915	0920	0925	0930	0935	0940	0945	0950	0955	ΣWIB	ΣTF
William Green	BCC	C	C	B	B	B	C	C	C	C	C	C	C	B	B	B	F	F	F	F	F	F	F	F	F	10	24
	WIB	-1	-1	+3	+1	+1	-1	-1	-1	-1	-1	-1	-3	+1	+1	+1	+1	+1	+1	+1	+1	+1	+3	+3	+1		
Edward James	BCC	P	V	A	A	A	A	E	B	O	O	A	A	A	A	P	F	F	F	F	F	F	B	B	A	57	21
	WIB	+3		+5	+5	+5	+5	+3	+1	+5	+1	+3	+3	+3	+3	+3	+1	+3	+3	+3	+1	+1	+1	+1	+3		
Minnie George	BCC	K	V	V	K	C	C	C	B	N	N	C	C	C	P	B	F	F	F	F	F	F	B	B	B	18	22
	WIB	+1			+1	-1	-1	-1	+1	+1	+1	-1	-1	-1	+1	+1	+1	+3	+3	+3	+1	+1	+1	+1			
Victor Coleman	BCC	K	K	W	K	C	C	C	K	P	C	K	B	B	K	K	P	F	L	F	F	F	B	N	N	16	24
	WIB	+1	+1	+1	+1	-1	-1	-1	+1	+1	-1	-1	+1	+1	-1	+1	+1	+1	+1	+1	+3	+3	+1	+1	+1		
Beatrice Quinlan	BCC	P	C	C	C	C	O	B	B	A	C	C	C	B	B	F	F	F	F	F	F	F	F	X	B	16	24
	WIB	+1	-1	-1	-1	-1	+1	+1	+1	+1	-1	-1	-1	+1	+1	-3	+1	+1	+3	+3	+3	+3	+1	+3	+1		

Date: 1.10.98 Time Period: 0955-1155 Place: No. Participants: 12 No. Staff: 3 + 1 agency Observer: Carole

Participant Name	Time	1000	1005	1010	1015	1020	1025	1030	1035	1040	1045	1050	1055	1100	1105	1110	1115	1120	1125	1130	1135	1140	1145	1150	1155	ΣWIB	ΣTF
William Green	BCC	F	F	N	C	N	B	N	N	N	C	C	B	F	F	C	N	N	C	C	B	B	X	V	V	12	22
	WIB	+1	+1	+1	-1	+1	+1	+1	+1	+1	-1	-1	+1	+1	+1	-1	+1	+1	-1	-1	+1	+1	+3				
Edward James	BCC	V	V	V	E	E	E	E	E	E	E	E	A	E	E	A	E	E	E	E	E	E	E	E	E	69	21
	WIB				+3	+3	+1	+5	+3	+5	+3	+5	+3	+3	+5	+3	+3	+3	+3	+3	+3	+3	+3	+3	+3		
Mnnie George	BCC	A	B	B	B	A	A	B	G	G	G	B	B	F	B	L	A	I	I	I	I	I	A	A	A	58	24
	WIB	+1	+1	+1	+1	+1	+1	+1	+5	+5	+5	+3	+1	+1	+1	+3	+3	+3	+3	+3	+3	+3	+3	+3	+3		
Victor Coleman	BCC	N	N	K	N	K	N	N	N	N	K	N	N	F	N	K	N	N	K	N	K	A	N	N	N	26	24
	WIB	+1	+1	+1	+1	+1	+1	+1	+1	+1	+1	+1	+1	+3	+1	+1	+1	+1	+1	+1	+1	+1	+1	+1	+1		
Beatrice Quinlan	BCC	A	B	A	B	B	I	I	I	I	I	B	B	F	I	I	I	I	I	I	I	I	A	A	A	53	23
	WIB	+1	+1	-1	+1	+1	+3	+3	+3	+3	+3	+1	+1	+1	+3	+3	+3	+3	+3	+3	+1	+3	+3	+3	+3		

Date: 1.10.98 Time Period: 1155-1355 Place: No. Participants: 12 No. Staff: 3 + 1 agency Observer: Carole

Participant Name	Time	1200	1205	1210	1215	1220	1225	1230	1235	1240	1245	1250	1255	1300	1305	1310	1315	1320	1325	1330	1335	1340	1345	1350	1355	ΣWIB	ΣTF
William Green	BCC	V	P	P	F	F	B	K	A	F	F	F	F	F	W	P	W	C	W	W	K	W	W	A	W	21	23
	WIB		+3	+1	+1	+1	+1	+1	+1	-1	-1	+3	+3	+3	-1	+3	+1	-1	+1	+1	-1	+1	+1	+1	+1		
Edward James	BCC	E	B	L	P	F	X	B	B	F	F	F	F	F	A	A	B	A	A	K	E	E	E	A	E	55	23
	WIB	+3	+1	+5		+1	+1	+1	+1	+3	+3	+3	+3	+3	+1	+3	+1	+3	+3	+3	+1	-3	+5	+3			
Minnie George	BCC	A	B	F	F	F	A	B	A	F	F	F	F	F	B	B	B	B	B	A	N	N	B	B	B	42	24
	WIB	+3	+1	+1	+1	+1	+3	+1	+1	+3	+3	+3	+3	+1	+1	+1	+1	+3	+3	+1	+1	+1	+1	+1			
Victor Coleman	BCC	P	B	A	B	B	M	B	M	F	F	F	F	F	B	A	N	N	N	N	B	B	N	N	N	26	24
	WIB	+3	+1	+3	+1	+1	+1	+1	+1	+3	+3	+3	+3	+3	+1	+3	-1	-1	-1	-1	+1	+1	-1	-1	-1		
Beatrice Quinlan	BCC	A	F	F	F	F	P	B	A	F	F	F	F	F	V	V	B	A	B	B	K	K	X	K	A	40	22
	WIB	+3	+1	+1	+1	+1	+1	+1	+1	+3	+3	+3	+3	+3			+1	+3	+1	+1	+1	+1	+3	+1	+3		

GUSHING OVER THEIR CARE

ENGLAND

CAROLINE BAKER describes a mapping exercise in Gloucestershire that was a really positive experience for all concerned, and which seemed to be part of a typical working day

I was asked to carry out an evaluation for an admission/assessment unit in Gloucester. I have asked the team there if it would be possible to share an extract of the map carried out as I feel it would make a significant contribution to our book of experiences, having left me without any doubt that person-centred care can be facilitated as an integral part of the 'normal working day' and become internalized within the staff if they are able to receive ongoing support and training.

It has been very difficult to extract two hours that would attempt to share the continual positive person work that was being carried out and indeed to try and convey my emotions on the day. I came away from the unit feeling thankful that DCM had been devised as I had been fortunate to be able to capture such good quality care and be able to feed back each and every positive moment to the staff, allowing them to reflect and understand just how much impact each and every member of the team had on improving people's well-being.

All of the staff team attended the feedback session and I can recall absolutely 'gushing' over the care that had been provided to a sea of faces that seemed unaware of their impact – which reaffirmed my belief that this did happen every day and not just because they were being evaluated on that particular day.

I would like to share two of the positive events with you, both of which relate to a gentleman many might consider 'extremely disabled', and who could so easily have been the subject of many Personal Detractions in a different environment. The gentleman concerned had a limited range of mobility and limited verbal communication skills. I began my observation at dinnertime. All the staff sat down and ate with the people they were caring for, laughing and socialising with them. I observed a member of staff sit down by the gentleman concerned and ask if he could cut up his food (which was on the plate) and the gentleman agreed. At this point, I was a little bemused as the gentleman was holding a spoon approximately 15cm from his mouth. I wondered how he was actually going to eat his lunch as he did not appear to make any attempt at

that time to move the spoon. The member of staff then placed some of the food onto his spoon, which the gentleman then manoeuvered to his mouth, ate the food and then pulled the spoon away again to the same position. I was overwhelmed that staff had both recognized and utilised this gentleman's abilities to the full and also allowed the time for this to occur, as this was recorded over a 35 minute period. So often, I have observed somebody in a similar situation being left in their chair in the lounge to be 'fed' by the care staff inside of 5 minutes.

The second situation occurred when the gentleman needed to move from the table to the toilet. He was consulted and prepared for the move and given time to listen to the staff's communication. Staff then walked either side of the gentleman, using a waist belt, completely in harmony with his every move, negotiating his next step and waiting patiently for his indication that he was ready to progress. Again, this event occurred over a 20 minute period and it could have been so easy for staff to place this gentleman in a wheelchair, as I believe he was when he was admitted.

I would like to thank all the staff at this unit for enabling me to witness such wonderful positive person work and person-centred care. It is a day that will stay with me for a very long time and continue to encourage me that the work we are doing does have such a valuable impact for people with dementia.

I can't say that any map has been a negative experience as I learn something from all of them, adapting my teaching and continuing to try and develop new ways of working with people with dementia. I do, however, struggle on occasions, when people are becoming obviously distressed and that distress is not being attended to. I confess that I intervene on most occasions either directly or to approach a member of staff, but then feed back to the staff what could have happened if I had not intervened.

The most common personal detractions I have recorded are objectification and disempowerment, usually mild or moderate in severity.

Being able to map is a privilege: to sit back and watch wonderful interactions between the people I am mapping, to observe great episodes of care and when it is not so good, and to be able to work with the staff to make a difference for the people we care for.

Date: June 2002   Time Period: 14.10 – 16.10   Place: --   No. Participants: 15   No. Staff: 5   Observer: CJB

Participant Name	Time	14.15	14.20	14.25	14.30	14.35	14.40	14.45	14.50	14.55	15.00	15.05	15.10	15.15	15.20	15.25	15.30	15.35	15.40	15.45	15.50	15.55	16.00	16.05	16.10	ΣWIB / ΣTF
1.	BCC	A	V	L	N	N	B	F	L	L	L	L	V	K	V	-	-	K	T	T	P	-	F	F	M	
	WIB	+1	-	+1	+1	+1	+1	+1	+1	+1	+1	+1		+3	Outside for a walk		+3	+3	+3	+3	+3	-	+1	+3	+3	
2.	BCC	B	B	A	K	K	F	F	F	B	K	K	B	K	V	-	-	K	B	F	F	-	V	-	-	
	WIB	+1	+1	+1	+3	+3	+3	+3	+1	+1	+1	+1	+1	+3	Outside for a walk		+3	+3	+3	+3	-	-	-	-	-	
3.	BCC	V	A	A	B	B	K	G	G	G	G	I	T	T	I	T	T	T	A	A	A	-	B	M	M	
	WIB	-	+1	+1	+1	+1	+3	+3	+3	+3	+3	+3	+3	+3	+1	+1	+1	+3	+3	+3	+3	-	+1	+3	+3	
4.	BCC	F	F	B	B	B	F	F	F	F	F	B	T	T	F	F	F	B	B	B	B	-	F	B	B	
	WIB	+3	+3	+1	+1	+1	+3	+3	+3	+3	+3	+3	+3	+3	+3	+3	+3	+3	+3	+3	+3	-	+3	+3	+3	
5.	BCC	T	T	T	A	A	A	A	A	A	T	A	A	A	A	A	A	A	T	T	M	-	K	F	K	
	WIB	+3	+3	+3	+3	+3	+3	+1	+1	+1	+3	+1	+1	+1	+3	+3	+3	+3	+3	+3	+1	-	+1	+1	+1	

Notes

- 14.30 Staff communicating with Participant 2 by writing things down as he is hard of hearing. **PE**
- 14.45 Participant 4 enjoying his cup of tea and marshmallows – he really smiled! Enjoying staff chatting to him.
- 14.55 Participant 1 clearing out her handbag
- 15.05 Participant 3 participating in a jigsaw

ENABLING EVIDENCE-BASED PRACTICE

AUSTRALIA

GAYLE HECKENBERG from Tasmania describes how she introduced DCM to a residential facility. She describes how the tool has enabled a move towards a more evidence-based approach to care

This map took place at Sandown Apartments, which is a low care residential facility with an 'ageing in place' philosophy.

The map was used as an information session for two staff members at management level to obtain an introduction to the mapping process. Previously I had spoken about DCM in formal settings, so the next step of showing staff practically gave them an overall picture of the data collection. The map highlighted important deficits in social interaction and Personal Detractions that influenced the behaviour of two residents that evening. The staff member caring for the residents received feedback on the mapping, and implementation of new strategies addressed the issues of concern.

The five residents mapped were in an evening group that is run from 4pm until 6pm every day of the week. Each resident is at a different stage of the dementing process and requires specifically designed activities within the group to address individual needs. Medical officers have written the diagnosis of dementia, but have not specified which type. Two out of the five residents have short-term memory loss but are capable of current conversation, the other three residents have both short and long-term memory loss, can converse but with prompting, and one resident out of these three speaks with jumbled words and unfinished sentences which you can see is very frustrating for her. All residents are female.

The map indicated to me the importance of the person-centred approach in identifying their well- and ill-being and the triggers that preceded certain patterns within their behaviour.

I saw very Positive Events taking place such as creative conversation, every individual receiving equity of time and obvious empathy and concern from the carer. However the Personal Detractors that I witnessed were infantilization and imposition. One resident became quite distressed in being forced to eat a sandwich that she did not want.

My best experience with mapping has been with the small group at Sandown where I have been able to re-map and identify the increased states of well-being, and more positive events than personal detractors. Previous strategies and interventions implemented as a result of mapping have clearly assisted the staff in their evaluation of issues that arise.

My worst experience was mapping in a facility where I witnessed disempowerment and infantilisation in its worst form at a lunchtime meal. The resident became so angry that she threw food across the table at the staff member and swore. The staff member had no idea that the approach she had taken had triggered this behaviour.

The most frequently recorded Personal Detractions I see are ignoring, infantilisation and disempowerment.

DCM has provided me with a tool that can measure quality services. It enables evidence-based practice and promotes person-centred care, allowing every individual to be seen as a unique entity. My mapping experience is limited, but I know that as it is embraced by others and my confidence is reinforced that the network within Australia and overseas will provide elderly people with the quality of care they so richly deserve.

Notes (see chart below)

- PB Mild (9) Carer not sensitive, but treating Flora and Dora as children.
- 1710 Carer forcing Flora to hold a sandwich which she did not want (mod 6)
- PE 1620 Stimulating very active interest in a game of cards – communicating very well with each resident

Date: 18.7.02	Time Period: 1600 - 1800	Place: Sandown Sundowners	No. Participants: 60	No. Staff: 7	Observer: G. Heckenberg

Participant Name	Time	1605	1610	1615	1620	1625	1630	1635	1640	1645	1650	1655	1700	1705	1710	1715	1720	1725	1730	1735	1740	1745	1750	1755	1800	ΣWIB / ΣTF
Molly	BCC	A	A	A	G	G	G	A	E	E	A	A	F	F	F	F	F	F	F	A	F	A	A	V	V	48
Molly	WIB	+1	+3	+3	+3	+3	+3	+3	+3	+3	+3	+3	+3	+1	+1	+1	+1	+1	+1	+1	+3	+1	+3	+3		22
Eve	BCC	A	A	A	E	E	A	A	N	N	A	B	F	F	F	F	F	F	A	A	A	A	A	L	L	42
Eve	WIB	+1	+1	+1	+3	+3	+1	+1	+1	+1	+1	+1	+1	+1	+3	+3	+1	+1	+1	+3	+3	+3	+3	+1	+1	24
Dora	BCC	A	A	A	G	G	G	G	G	A	A	L	L	F	F	F	F	F	A	A	A	B	B	P	P	52
Dora	WIB	+1	+3	+3	+3	+3	+3	+3	+3	+3	+3	+3	+3	+3	+3	+3	+1	+1	+1	+1	+1	+1	+1	+1	+1	24
Doris	BCC	B	B	A	A	G	G	G	L	L	L	L	F	F	F	F	F	F	F	F	A	B	B	A	V	33
Doris	WIB	+1	+1	+1	+3	+1	+1	+1	+3	+3	+3	+3	+1	+1	+1	+1	+1	+1	+1	+1	+1	+1	+1	+1	+1	23
Flora	BCC	B	B	C	C	C	N	N	N	B	B	B	A	F	F	F	F	A	A	F	F	F	F	B	B	18
Flora	WIB	+1	+1	-1	-1	-1	+1	+1	+1	+1	+1	+1	+1	+1	+1	+1	+1	+1	+1	+1	+1	+1	+1	+1	+1	23

'WE COULD HAVE DONE WITH A STATISTICIAN!'

SCOTLAND

GERRY MONTGOMERY & MERVYN GRANGER describe how they used dementia care mapping in Dumbarton. They use mapping as an audit tool to evaluate developing person-centred care

We are community psychiatric nurses whose specific remit is in dementia. We carry out home assessments as part of our duties as well as providing support and advice to others, eg carers, relatives and other professionals. We co-ordinate packages of care involving regular joint working with a range of care providers.

We are based at Dumbarton Joint Hospital, which is in Central Scotland. The area we cover is a mixture of small urban patches and larger rural patches. We did our basic DCM training in June 2002 and carried out our first mapping in September 2002. All in we did a total of 40 hours over a period of 5 days in a fortnight.

It took place in a local 12 bedded NHS continuing care unit for people with dementia. The unit opened one year ago and the manager wished an evaluation to be carried out after the first year. The residents are all continuing care with a primary diagnosis of a dementia, who present with challenging behaviours.

The results are to be used as an audit tool to evaluate the success of the person-centred care approach which was adopted as the care philosophy when the unit first opened. The results indicate that the overall culture of the unit fit into the 'new' culture suggested in the 7th Edition of the DCM Manual (p88).

Our best experience mapping was being able to see first hand the approach of very caring and skilled individuals in their interactions with the residents, and the success of those interactions. Also, we were received by staff and residents alike in a very positive way throughout.

Our worst experience was analysing the results! We could have done with a full time statistician. In all honesty, though, it was a truly remarkable experience and it was a privilege to be part of the care environment albeit for a small period of time.

Date: 9/9/02 Time Period: 0900-1100 Place: No. Participants: 12 No. Staff 5 Observers: Gerry Montgomery

Participant Name	Time	0905	0910	0915	0920	0925	0930	0935	0940	0945	0950	0955	1000	1005	1010	1015	1020	1025	1030	1035	1040	1045	1050	1055	1100	ΣWIB / ΣTF
1	BCC	F	F	F	F	K	K	A	C	A	C	T	T	K	A	K	V	V	A	P	K	V	A	F	B	+25
	WIB	+1	+1	+3	+1	-1	-1	+1	-1	+1	-1	+1	+1	+1	+3	+1		+3	+3	+1		+5	+1	+1		21
2	BCC	F	P	F	F	F	F	B	B	A	P	P	P	P	T	B	N	N	B	N	A	P	B	F	P	+32
	WIB	+1	+1	+1	+3	+1	+1	+1	+1	1	+3	+3	+1	+1	+1	+1	+1	+1	+1	+1	+1	+1	+1	+3	+1	24
3	BCC	M	M	F	F	M	A	M	M	X	M	M	M	M	M	M	M	M	V	V	M	M	F	M	M	+59
	WIB	+3	+3	+1	+3	+3	+3	+3	+3		+3	+3	+3	+3	+3	+3	+3	+3			+3	+3	+1	+3	+3	21
	BCC																									
	WIB																									
	BCC																									
	WIB																									

'YOU DON'T HAVE TO SAY YES BECAUSE YOU'VE BEEN ASKED'

ENGLAND

HAZEL MAY shows us a map that formed part of a review into standards of care for social services purchasers. The map describes a range of positive events and personal detractors

This map is taking place in a residential home in England. The results will be used to inform purchasers about 'best value' in their area and to improve services in nursing and residential care for the future. I have been called in as an independent, external researcher and so I know very little about the people being mapped except that they live in a long term care setting, and they have dementia.

I see in the map some very strong, resourceful people who have dementia: people who have a strong drive to live and to have an impact on the world around them. I also see staff working hard but struggling because of their limited knowledge and experience regarding the special needs of people with dementia. There is nobody there to help them while they work or to show them possibilities for improving their own or residents' well-being.

My best experience using DCM was some years ago in a Saturday Club, newly opened for people with dementia. A great deal of thought and care had been invested into the development of this service. Despite the environment being rather small and 'hospital-like', the experience of being there for clients and staff was fantastic. It felt very rewarding to be able to map what many people believe to be the unachievable.

My worst experience of DCM was in a private organisation where the care was very poor. The results of the map showed this and, although the staff themselves were keen to move forward and make improvements, the owner of the nursing home was angry. He put me down and rubbished the whole method in front of all the staff and I had to work really hard not to burst into tears and run out. He thought that 'buying in' DCM would make his home look attractive. I learned a lot from this experience about the importance of in-depth preparatory work in the lead up to a project. And that you don't always have to say 'yes' just because you've been asked.

The personal detractors that I map most frequently are, without a doubt, ignoring and objectification.

Participant Name		Time Frame 12.05	12.10	12.15	12.20	12.25	12.30	12.35	12.40	12.45	12.50	12.55	1.00	1.05	1.10	1.15	1.20	1.25	1.30	1.35	1.40	1.45	1.50	1.55	2.00	ΣWIB / ΣTF
Elsie	BCC	A	B	K	K	K	K	K	B	P	K	F	F	F	F	F	F	F	F	F	F	F	K	M	M	
	WIB	+1	+1	+1	+1	+1	+3	+1	+1	+1	+1	+1	+1	+1	+1	+1	+1	+1	+1	+1	+1	+1	+1	+3	+3	+3
Phillipa	BCC		B	F	F	F	F	F	F	F	F	F	F	F	F	F	F	F	F	F	F	A	A	A	A	
	WIB		+1	+1	-1	+3	+3	+1	+3	+3	+1	+1	+1	+1	+1	+1	+1	+1	+1	+1	+1	+5	+3	+3	+5	
Celia	BCC	N	N	C	C	N	C	C	A	P		F	F	F	F	B	B	F	C	C	F	P	B	B	N	
	WIB	+1	+1	-1	-1	+1	-1	-1	+1	+1		-1	+1	+1	-1	+1	+1	-1	-1	-1	+3	+1	+1	+1	+1	
Maggie	BCC	C	K		K	D	C	N	N	F	F	F	F	F	F	F	K	V	V	V	V	V	V	V	L	
	WIB	-1	+1		+1	+1	-1	+1	+1	+1	+3	+3	+1	+3	+1	-1	+1	V	V	V	V	V	V	V	+1	
Jane	BCC			C	C	C	Y	A	A		P	F	F	F	B	A	A		A	F	A	B	B	A	B	B	B	
	WIB			-1	-1	-1	+1	+1	+1	+3	+3	+1	+1	+1	+1	+1	+3	+1	+1	+1	+1	+3	+1	+1	+1	

Notes

- Maggie has a Yorkshire terrier dog on her lap. Jane is much younger than anybody else, in her early 50s.
- 12.07 **PD** 'She's just wet her slippers if you are wondering where they are.'
- A lady in the sitting area chunters on about young people today and sings occasionally.
- 12.09 care worker appears and takes food away from the lady next to Phillipa and gives it to Phillipa who starts to eat it. The other lady joins in, eating from Phillipa's plate with her fingers before pulling the plate away from Phillipa.
- 12.15 Lady in the lounge calls out 'don't let them shut me in please, please don't...' Phillipa tries to retrieve her food 'Oi, c'm

'ere' Jane walks to the table and stands looking at the plate of food, Phillipa moves herself away in her chair.

- **PD** care worker arrives 'hello sexy how ya doin'?'

'Doris, what are you doing eating Phillipa's lunch?'

- **PD** The care worker proceeds to pick up the bowl and spoon feed Phillipa.
- **PD** She turns to the other residents and says 'If you're picking up droppings, you've got a long wait' and then to Phillipa 'You steamy sex pot you. Have you accosted Will yet? I've just had a punch up in the bathroom' (this goes on with care worker calling Phillipa 'sexy' and 'luvvy'.
- **PD** Two care workers chat while helping residents with their lunch 'I've just caught her eating Phillipa's lunch' 'Yes, that's about right, she'll eat everyone else's but not her own'

- 12.25 Maggie takes food out of her mouth and throws it against the wall (as If it's hard, like nuts?) Phillipa enjoys one-to-one attention from care worker who is spoon feeding her.
- 12.28 **PD** 'You're going to have to learn to sit down at lunch time otherwise the puppy dog will have your food; are you off with the flowers again luvvy?'
- **PD** two care workers chat making reference to 'battling Bill' who has 'contaminated the bathroom' and 'piddled up the wall'
- 12.30 Elsie enjoys attention from care worker.
- 12.33 Elsie sits in care worker's chair, hovering over the plate of food
- **PD** She is reprimanded loudly and publicly by care worker as if she were a naughty child 'Elsie that's not yours'
- 12.40 **PD** (re Phillipa) 'Is she not feeding herself?' 'No' – see note at 12.09!! Phillipa can feed herself.
- 12.43 **PD** Objectification, medication popped into Elsie's mouth – just like posting a letter.
- **PD** 'Did Constance get toileted? She's gonna have to be fed today, she's on antibiotics'
- 12.45 Phillipa now holding her own drink.
- **PD** care worker (to Jane) 'Janey, lunch time' 'Ooh' says Jane. Two care workers mimic her 'ooh' and laugh. (Identifying infantilisation and mockery)
- **PD** Maggie is feeding her dog from the table 'MAGGIE NO' shouts a care worker extremely loudly 'IT'S YOUR FOOD' – Maggie replies 'It pleases me if I feed her or put it up the wall.' Maggie makes Jane laugh
- **PD** care worker literally 'stuffs' food with her fingers into Jane's mouth in a very rushed fashion.
- **PD** care worker tries to hurt the dog, he reaches under the table to get the dog but the dog retaliates by snapping at him. So does Maggie saying 'I woudn't have you for my brother'. 'You're 93' replies the care worker in a condescending tone. Jane tries to leave and Celia says she doesn't want her lunch but another care worker sits quietly helping her.
- Maggie flicks food intermittently at the care worker who hurt her dog (the dog has fled!)

- **PD** Elsie is eating independently but a care worker comes and takes her knife and fork from her and cuts up her food for her. The care worker returns to Jane who makes a noise, which he mimics back at her. 'Elsie, have you got your teeth in, I don't think so' he says.
- 1.10 **PD** care worker sits down to eat his own lunch leaning over to put bread and butter into Elsie's mouth while she is still eating.
- 1.11 **PD** Another care worker asks 'has everyone eaten OK?' and colleague responds 'Elsie has eaten very slowly – she hasn't got her teeth.' 'Aha' comes the reply 'look what I've found.' care worker proceeds to put Elsie's teeth into her mouth and gives her a drink 'That's better, you look much more like my Elsie now.' The conversation continues 'She (Maggie) has been throwing food at me, I caught her feeding Angus (the dog) and she got cross' Celia is chewing miserably with her head in her hands, Maggie looks upset.
- 1.20 **PD** care worker takes knife out of Elsie's hand and takes over her feeding saying in a sarcastic tone 'we usually use a spoon or a fork for that kind of operation.'
- 1.30 **PD** Two care workers chat while they feed people 'Has her chest been checked out?' 'Well, she smoked about 40 a day so she's always been rattly' (He did go on to say that he would arrange further checks if there was no improvement in a couple of days)
- 'Elsie's eaten all her custard and jam and left the tart'
- 'I'm going to get everyone a drink, are you going to help me Jane or are you going to just sit there... Ok, just sit there' (care worker cross with Jane)
- 1.40 Celia gives care worker a kiss in gratitude for her drink.
- 1.45 Phillipa's daughter arrives.
- 1.52 Elsie enjoys one-to-one attention from care worker who then gives her a book to look at. She turns the pages and looks interested.
- 1.57 Phillipa is holding hands with her daughter looking very happy.

REFLECTING ON PERSONAL PRACTICE

ENGLAND

JUNIPER WEST & JUDITH FARMER, based in Norfolk, describe how the process of DCM has enabled them to reflect on their practice and develop person-centred care

I completed the Bradford University run Dementia Care Mapping Course (Basic) in April 2002 and have had the opportunity to map on about three occasions. The first two were by myself; the third was with an experienced mapper, Judith. It is this third 'practice' map that we are writing about today.

This map took place on the ward on which I work, therefore the people we were mapping were very familiar to me, but not to Judith. The aims primarily today were for me to practise mapping with someone else experienced, rather than specifically for ward feedback. This was also in preparation for a large mapping project I was to be involved with within our directorate. The ward staff were briefed beforehand that today's aim was just that. The map lasted for approximately two hours, by the time we had sorted out whom we were going to map and how we were going to work together.

We chose four people to map but added another 'in reserve' to observe in case someone was taken off the ward for therapy activity during the mapping period. We mapped from 09.55 to 11.50, four women and one man. For the purposes of this report, the names have been replaced with numbers.

1. Is a lady who has recently suffered a major stroke following a hip replacement operation, which is causing her difficulties with mobility. She also experiences severe dysphasia. She has been living alone in a country village with lots of family support and has been staying on the ward for about a month. The team is concerned about her low mood. She sits with her head in her hands and experiences periods of frustration and anger. She can mobilise independently with a frame.

2. Is a lady who has been on the ward for some time (since May) and has been living in care for several years. She is a widow with minimal contact with her family. She has a history of depression going back to 1995 for which she received treatment in hospital. She can be independently

mobile but generally sits for long periods. She very rarely speaks.

3. Is a gentleman who has been living at home with his wife but who had to be compulsorily admitted to hospital. He experiences some deafness at a distance.

4. Is a lady who has been staying on the ward for two months. During this time, her husband died suddenly at home. He was her main carer. But her son is also very supportive. She has a two-three year history of leaving her home and being unable to recognise where she is.

5. Is a lady who has been admitted to hospital in the last few days and transferred to us from another ward just yesterday. She is experiencing difficulty with mobility and uses a frame.

The period that we were mapping was during a fairly quiet time on the ward, where everyone was sitting down after the hustle and bustle of getting up, dressed and eating breakfast. We are aware that the data gathered is over too short a period to accurately reflect the overall behaviour and well-being of individuals and this group.

The group spent 61% of time in behaviour categories B and N. The WIB score for the group is +1.0.

There were few signs of ill-being and the impression was of a group quietly sitting and observing any activity. This showed in the data. It included the potential for each person to engage with others and to increase their well-being.

My best experience with DCM has been the opportunity to sit, away from the ward work, and reflect on my own practice as well as recognise potential opportunities for positive interventions. It is a huge learning experience to increase your sense of empathy for individuals with dementia.

My worst experience was actually working on a ward that was being mapped. I remember feeling extremely self-conscious and aware of my working practices. On reflection this was a valuable learning and self-awareness exercise too. (Juni)

The best experience for me (Judith) has definitely been when working as a team leader in a day hospital and using mapping to introduce a person-centred approach and then as part of the team development over a two-year period. The worst experience has been when I have used mapping as a one-off exercise without working alongside a team.

Date: 13.9.02   Time Period: 0950 - 1200   Place: --   No. Participants: x4   No. Staff: x5   Observer: Judith Farmer/Juniper West

Participant Name		Time	09.55	10.00	10.05	10.10	10.15	10.20	10.25	10.30	10.35	10.40	10.45	10.50	10.55	11.00	11.05	11.10	11.15	11.20	11.25	11.30	11.35	11.40	11.45	11.50	ΣWIB / ΣTF
1	BCC		N	N	N	-	K	B	B	F	F	F	C	C	C	K	B	B	B	K	O	C	C	K	B	O	13
	WIB		+1	+1	+1	-	+1	+1	+1	+1	+1	+1	-1	-1	-1	+1	+1	+1	+1	+1	+1	-1	-1	+1	+1	+1	23
2	BCC		N	N	N	-	N	N	N	N	P	N	P	N	N	N	N	N	N	N	N	N	N	N	N	N	23
	WIB		+1	+1	+1	-	+1	+1	+1	+1	+1	+1	+1	+1	+1	+1	+1	+1	+1	+1	+1	+1	+1	+1	+1	+1	23
3	BCC					-		B		F	F	O	N	N	X	O	B	N	B	B	N	K	B	B	B	B	18
	WIB					-		+1		+1	+1	+1	+1	+1	+1	+1	+1	+1	+1	+1	+1	+1	+1	+1	+1	+1	18
4	BCC		A	A	A	-	A	A	X	P								P	/	A	A	A	A	A	A	A	16
	WIB		+1	+1	+1	-	+1	+1	+1	+1								+1	/	+1	+3	+1	+1	+1	+1		14
5	BCC		B	B	B	-	B	B	B	B	F	F	B	B	B	A	B	P	B	B	B	B	B	B	B	B	27
	WIB		+1	+1	+1	-	+1	+1	+1	+1	+1	+1	+1	+3	+1	+1	+1	+3	+1	+1	+1	+1	+1	+1	+1	+1	23

Notes

- 10.05 Reduced staff activity in the lounge – one visit from care worker
- 10.23 Participant 3 looking a bit perplexed/anxious – walked up to his room hesitantly and alone.
- 10.40 Care worker gently woke Participant 5, at eye level; offered tea, helped to sit up but elicited only opening eyes.
- 10.40 Participant 4 went to occupational therapy group.
- 10.50 Jessie looking over several times as though wishing to talk – two care workers present.
- 11.10 Participant 5 expressing feelings about her predicament to physios, and clearly appreciating this.

A GOOD VIEWPOINT ON DEMENTIA CARE

JAPAN

KATSUYA YAMAMOTO offers a Japanese perspective, from Nagoya. DCM is used to evaluate care and develop cost-effective, caring services. The data describes a range of positive events and PDs

I have been mapping for half a year, at a geriatric health services facility and special nursing home for elderly people. We use mapping to provide better quality facilities for people with dementia, and to help reform long-term care insurance in Japan.

Dementia Care Mapping gives me a good viewpoint on dementia care and helps form better relationships with caregivers. My understanding of dementia care is better then before.

My only negative comments are that the time frame of 5 minutes is very long, in that staff are always near the patients in our facility.

Notes

14.05–14.10 **PE** Some staff greeted Yoshikawa when they walk near her table

14.10–14.15 **PE** When Yoshikawa said she had bad condition, staff took her hands and asked the condition

14.20–14.25 **PD** Yoshikawa didn't watch video, but some staff made her watch it

14.35–14.40 **PE** When some staff gave Yoshikawa a drink and she gave one to her doll too

14.30–14.35 **PE** Staff took Umemiya to the room's toilet with talking friendly and joyful

14.50–55 **PE** Staff brought out Kuni's topic for her favourite colour using tea time sweets

14.10–14 **PE** When Saito was angry with somebody's abusive words and excited, staff didn't miss that and made contact

15.40–45 Yamamoto went upstairs with staff to get toilet paper

15.10–15 **PD** Staff blamed Yamamoto's failure of forgetting some promise

15.25–30 **PD** Staff presented many choices

16.05–10 **PE** When Yamamoto was crying, staff gave pretty straw hat using Japanese traditional dance

---

Date: Sept 2002 Time Period: 13.55 – 15.00 Place: No. Participants: 3 No. Staff: 4 Observer: KY

Participant Name	Time	14.00	14.05	14.10	14.15	14.20	14.25	14.30	14.35	14.40	14.45	14.50	14.55	15.00										ΣWIB / ΣTF
Yoshikawa	BCC	A	K	A	K	A	A	A	B	K	M	F	A											
	WIB	+1	+3	+5	+3	+1	+1	+1	+3	+1	-1	+3												
Irino	BCC	Q	M	W	B	N	N	W	A	N	N	W	F											
	WIB	+1	-1	+1	+1	+1	+1	-1	-1	+1	+1	-1												
Umemiya	BCC	M	M	M	M	M	X	M	M	M	M	M	M											
	WIB	+3	+3	+3	+3	+3	-3	+3	+3	+1	+1	+1												

Date: Sept 2002 Time Period: 14.00 – 15.00 Place: No. Participants: 3 No. Staff: 4 Observer: KY

Participant Name	Time	14.00	14.05	14.10	14.15	14.20	14.25	14.30	14.35	14.40	14.45	14.50	14.55	15.00										ΣWIB / ΣTF
Kuni	BCC	E	E	E	X	X	E	E	E	E	E	F	A											
	WIB	+5	+5	+3	+1	+1	+1	+1	+3	+3	+3	+3	+3											
Saito	BCC	A	X	A	A	A	A	A	G	A	A	A	B											
	WIB	+3	+5	+3	+3	+3	+3	+1	+5	+1	+1	+1	+1											
Yamamoto	BCC	A	A	C	C	A	J	A	A	A	A	A	F											
	WIB	-3	+1	-1	-1	-1	-1	-1	-1	-1	-1	-1	-1											

Date:		Time Period: 15.10 – 16.05				Place:		No. Participants: 3				No. Staff:										Observer:	
Participant Name	Time	15.10	15.15	15.20	15.25	15.30	15.35	15.40	15.45	15.50	15.55	16.00	16.05										ΣWIB / / ΣTF	
Kuni	BCC	A	A	A	A	A	B	B	B	B	B	B	B											
	WIB	+5	+3	+3	+3	+3	+3	+3	+3	+3	+3	+3	+3											
Saito	BCC	A	A	N	A	B	A	A	A	A	A													
	WIB	+1	+1	+1	+1	+1	+1	+1	+1	+1	+1													
Yamamoto	BCC	F	A	A	A	A	A		L	C	A	X												
	WIB	-1	-1	-3	-1	-3	-1		+1	-3	+1	+1												

Date: Aug 2002		Time Period: 15.30 – 16.30					Place:		No. Participants: 3		No. Staff: 4			Observer: KY										
Participant Name	Time	15.30	15.35	15.40	15.45	15.50	15.55	16.00	16.05	16.10	16.15	16.20	16.25	16.30									ΣWIB / / ΣTF	
Ito	BCC	F	L	L	L	L	L	L	N	A	L													
	WIB	+1	+3	+3	+3	+3	+3	+3	+1	-3	+5													
Kurimura	BCC	F	F	F	A	A	A	B	A	B	A	L	L											
	WIB	+1	+1	+1	+3	+3	-1	+1	-1	+1	+3	+1	+1											
Shida	BCC	F	F	L	K	B	B	B	A	B	B	B	B											
	WIB	+1	+1	+1	+1	+3	+1	+1	+1	+1	+1	+1	+1											

THE THURSDAY CLUB

ENGLAND

LISA HELLER presents a profound insight into a day centre facility known as the Thursday Club. She used mapping to demonstrate the effectiveness of the service the club provided

In June of this year, I had the good fortune to map a day centre, called "The Thursday Club". It was an experience I shall cherish, as I watched and joined in with a club where everyone treated everyone else as equals. There was friendship, fun, wonderful food, prepared by a group of people whose ages ranged from seventeen to ninety, and some magical moments of skilled care. The club is run by the Alzheimer's Society, and is attended by eight people, all living in the local area, some alone, and others with their carer. But a crisis was looming – it had been proposed that the local authority would cease to fund the club, after fifteen years. This was an unusual map in my experience, in that it was possible to see important elements of person-centred care firmly in place. While I was there, I pondered the development of the theory of 'relationship centred care'. So much of what happened here was possible because of the relationships which were built and sustained between attenders and the workers who cared for them.

The map of the Thursday Club had been planned for some time, but when the organisation heard that their funding was threatened, they asked for the map to be done straight away, as they hoped that it might help in their efforts to secure their future.

So the results of the map were important to the staff in two ways. They wished to consider ways of improving the care they give, and also they hoped the report would add weight to their efforts to keep the centre open. Three out of the seven regular staff are trained mappers; all have attended sessions on Person Centred Care.

The main things which the staff team asked the mappers to consider were:
• Any bad habits they might have fallen into without realising
• The beginnings and endings of the days
• Three participants who cause concern:
– Jack, who tends to close his eyes, and disengage from what is going on.
– Eva, who tends to look after Gina, who seeks her out. Is this her choice?
– Tom, who has limited verbal communication and tends to use sarcasm and jokiness. How is it best to respond to him?

Two briefing sessions were held, and handouts on DCM given to staff. My co-mapper and I visited the club and got to know people. We conducted an Inter-rater Reliability test and then set the dates for the full map.

The map was conducted over two days, so we collected about eight full hours of data on each attender.

Two days after the map, all care workers were given a short written initial feedback summary, when the first data processing had been done. A meeting was arranged for the following day to allow them to discuss anything which had arisen, either from the experience of mapping, or from the feedback so far.

Then, ten days later, a full feedback meeting was arranged. All the care workers involved attended these meetings, and engaged with the feedback. Among the things which were said were, "It makes you think, doesn't it. There are things which you might never have thought of if you didn't let someone outside observe what goes on."

We commented on the issues that they had asked us to consider.

First, any bad habits? We thought there might be a tendency to be slightly patronising in verbal tone on occasion. One of the two Personal Detractions we recorded was infantilisation. Staff acknowledged that this sometimes happened, and the worker responsible voluntarily identified himself. A discussion followed as to why this might happen. The worker concerned and others felt that it was a valid recording. They thought that this tendency arose because they were constantly working to keep the mood of the group high, using jokes and banter. We wondered if this care worker used this kind of banter in his usual contacts with people?

Secondly, the end of the day. Each attender goes home with a copy of a brief summary of the day. We commented on the routine of leaving the writing of the summaries until the last minute, so that home time was a bit more rushed and fraught than it might have been. Having said that, the attenders were familiar with the reason for this, and seemed content to wait patiently. It was suggested that attenders might like to be involved with writing their daily record. Some wanted this record for themselves, others said they would be giving it to their carer.

Apart from this, we were impressed by the confident way in which attenders waited for their turn on the transport. What might have been an anxious time was generally calm, sociable and productive.

In discussion about our observation of the three attenders who gave cause for concern, the staff were interested to see what had been observed, and to listen to our thoughts and suggestions. The team resolved to try and continue to observe what the attenders concerned really seemed to want, and to try to work with them to enable them to have the best day that they could. It was acknowledged that, although it was generally a very happy and lively day, some people might feel unhappy or uncomfortable at times. If this is recognised, workers can allow people to express their feelings and help them to feel validated.

One lady stood out as an example of the group for me. A

small lady with a neat pleated skirt and a brooch at her collar, Janie entered the room like a bird, talking, moving quickly, and darting her eyes round to see who was there and what was happening. She sat near to me, and waited to be introduced. She wanted to know about me, and why I was there, and we briefly chatted about what might happen during the day. Later, Janie chose from a range of knives and peelers offered to her, and helped to make vegetable soup. She found the caretaker, and asked him to play the piano whilst she danced in the corridor. She carried dirty cups to the kitchen and helped to wash and dry them. She offered me lunch and drinks when she could see that these were on their way, and she walked in the garden, picking a few flowers. She joined in with everything and she sang or whistled most of the time. She carried on a kind of running commentary on the day, noticing when something new was about to start, exclaiming with pleasure, "Oh, we're going to have a cup of tea now, there will be buns!" She in fact acted as if she belonged – even as if she owned the place.

Her need for someone who she knew and trusted was apparent at times – she would look up and see a strange face, and immediately stop what she was doing, searching for someone familiar. As soon as she was reassured, by a word or a touch, from someone she knew, she resumed her cheerful occupation.

The staff worked with and alongside Janie and the other attenders, enabling them, providing opportunities, recognising attachment needs, and enjoying moments of playful laughter together. Everyone here belonged, there was no question about anyone's membership of the club.

Date: 12.7.02   Time Period: 10.20 – 12.20   Place: No. Participants: 8   No. Staff: 5   Observer: Lisa Heller

Name		10.25	10.30	10.35	10.40	10.45	10.50	10.55	11.00	11.05	11.10	11.15	11.20	11.25	11.30	11.35	11.40	11.45	11.50	11.55	12.00	12.05	12.10	12.15	12.20	ΣWIB / ΣTF
Janie Cotteshaw	BCC	F	F	A	E	L	M	M	M	L	V	L	L	L	L	L	L	L	L	L	K	A	T	T	A	68
	WIB	+3	+1	+3	+1	+3	+3	+3	+3	+3		+3	+3	+5	+5	+3	+5	+3	+3	+3	+3	+3	+3	+3	+3	22
Jack Wilson	BCC	F	A	F	B	O	X	F	B	M	A	A	K	T	T	A	P	T	A	A	A	J	A	B	E	62
	WIB	+3	+3	+3	+1	+1	+3	+3	+1	+1	+3	+3	+3	+3	+3	+3	+3	+3	+3	+3	+3	+3	+3	+1	+3	24
Eva Brookes	BCC	A	F	F	A	M	A	A	M	M	M	M	M	X	K	V	A	A	A	A	A	J	B	A	E	69
	WIB	+5	+3	+3	+3	+3	+3	+3	+3	+3	+3	+3	+3	+1	+3		+3	+3	+3	+3	+3	+3	+3	+3	+3	23
Gina Weston	BCC	A	A	F	F	A	A	A	A	A	K	L	L	L	L	L	A	T	A	V	P	P	A	M	M	69
	WIB	+3	+3	+3	+3	+3	+1	+3	+3	+3	+3	+3	+3	+3	+3	+3	+3	+3		+3	+3	+3	+5	+3		23
Tom Ellwood	BCC			A	A	F	A	A	A/	A	A	A	P	P	P	O	O	K	K	K	K	T	J	J		68
	WIB			+3	+3	+3	+3	+3	+3	+3	+3	+3	+3	+3	+3	+3	+3	+3	+3	+5	+5	+3	+3	+3	+3	21

Notes

10.25 Eva complimented on her outfit – much laughter as she showed it off with a twirl, and talked about how her daughter wanted her to buy a new one – "This is an old thing from upstairs".

Attenders greeted care worker making toast in the corner.

10.40 Janie wants to be busy, humming to herself, then gets up to clear away.

10.50 **PE** Jack helped to toilet.

Care worker shows copies of photos she has borrowed. Janie and Eva's weddings, small children etc. Gina very interested.

Tom needing reassurance, anxious about going home. Care worker, sitting close by him, holds his hand and chats.

11.00 Tom asking about mappers.

11.10 Jack moved on invitation of care worker to be nearer to care worker and involved in looking at photos, chatting. [Attachment, Validation]

11.15 Tom offered painting, agreed, small table set up.

Walk across garden to church offered. Pat, Jim and Teresa to go with two care workers (Charlie and Fiona)

11.20 Tom not wanting to paint, nails cleaned and cut instead.

11.35 Tom finishes job off, tidying himself as well. With two care workers.

11.45 Tom joined in chat. Walking round with care workers watching through window.

Flowers brought in from walk, shown and smelt.

11.55 Janie helps with lunch – she's humming while she works.

12.05 Jack, Eva and Tom all play wth soft ball.

12.10 Takes honeysuckle to smell.

NO LONGER LEFT UNATTENDED

AUSTRALIA

MARGARET RANDALL from New South Wales explains how she used the data from her mapping to work with a staff team to develop ways of improving person-centred care

I began to map at Allandale Aged Care Facility. Guided by Dr Kim Wylie I soon learned some of the finer details of mapping, and I am still learning after forty-nine hours of mapping. In August, accompanied by the Director of Nursing, Marolyn Seaman, I mapped for the first time at this care facility.

The facility has a dementia specific unit. It accommodates ten residents and has a full time staff of two assistants in nursing (AIN) with a registered nurse readily available. I work within this unit for four two-hour periods per week as a diversional therapist, providing a range of activities to improve residents' well-being. Residents are free to participate. No attempt is made to coerce them into group or individual programs. Sometimes all ten residents join in. At other times there may be one or two. The AINs, while attending to the residents' personal care needs, are involved in activities too. Our aim is for each resident to experience meaningful engagement with their social and physical environment throughout their day.

DCM Education

When the unit first opened, intensive in-service was provided for staff and this program is ongoing. However, DCM is seen to be a means of continuous quality improvement through developmental evaluation. Hence, on Friday 26 July 2002, the first DCM in-service program was held. It was organised for an hour before and after change of shifts to give all those who worked in the Armstrong Wing a chance to attend. Perhaps the biggest impact from this session was the fact that staff could see DCM held the potential to capture the many satisfying and enjoyable events which happened in a resident's daily life. It would be a means of 'keeping track' of such events in a way that current documentation failed to do. The initial program explored the concept of a 'person-centred approach' and the use of DCM as a means of developmental evaluation. We briefly touched on 'personal detractors' and positive event records.

The next DCM education program was offered on 12 August at the same time to enable all staff concerned to attend. This session was taped so that all those who missed out could view it at a later date. During the session methods for collecting and recording data were explained. Staff were somewhat mesmerised by the coding frames for behaviour until it was explained that the DCM manual was a constant companion during a mapping session.

The mapping on 15 August was probably the hardest mapping which I had undertaken. One of the residents was

dying and her family was there with her. This lady had endeared herself to both staff and residents and it was not easy to sit as an observer and sense the grief that these people were experiencing.

The feedback to staff occurred on Monday 2 September. Again the feedback session was offered in two sessions and was also videotaped. This was a very interesting and interactive experience for all. The main overheads used were the 'behaviour category grid' and the Individual WIB Profiles.

Those present found it interesting to see how the residents had spent their time while we were mapping. Despite the sombre mood in the unit there had been some meaningful involvement. The percentages of time coded 'cool or withdrawn' and 'sleep' were down on each of my previous mapping sessions in other places.

We looked at Mollie's individual WIB scores. The question arose, "How does one respond to the needs of residents who are experiencing grief?" Mollie had become a comforter of Emily during their day-to-day living. She was often seen in Emily's room holding her hand and gently talking to her at times when Emily was somewhat distressed. Certainly Mollie was not being neglected. However the hugs and cuddles and words of comfort that Mollie was receiving were not long enough to be coded with positive WIB scores, rather she was left alone for much of the time to wander the corridor outside Emily's room or sit alone in the dining room. Only on the occasions when firstly an AIN, and later a relative of Emily came to take her in to Emily, was Mollie's grief responded to. But, towards the end of the mapping a AIN invited Mollie to join the group for a game of dominoes. Such was the change in Mollie's well-being that this ten-minute period was coded with two +3s. She joined in the conversation and laughter – coded A +3, and enjoyed the game – coded G +3.

Personal Detractions in this mapping included PD7a (Outpacing) – "Where's Lilly/come this way/turn right" and "I've got some lovely fruit for you. Where do you want to sit – lounge or here?" and PD2a (Disempowerment) "No, sit here". PD13a (Withholding) – Mollie spent much of the two-hour period preoccupied by her concern for Emily. Staff did not respond to her need until the last ten minutes when she was included in the domino game. (On the other hand they did try – took her in to see Emily and gave her hugs and cuddles.)

Dealing with grief was seen as one area of concern for staff. During the discussion they said that it is not only the residents who feel the loss of someone who had lived with them and to whom they had become attached. One suggestion was that there be more education about dealing with grief. Some even suggested that this would help them to cope with the 'loss' of a resident who is transferred elsewhere when their need for more care was evident.

Responding to grief is already part of the in-service training at the unit and there is also a video. But staff felt it would be better to have an interactive type of program.

The game of dominoes attracted other comments too. The nurse guiding the residents was obviously not familiar with the concept of dementia. She repeatedly told Alice to 'think' before she placed a domino. This made Alice become more and more agitated: a dressmaker in her day, she began to rub the tablecloth and pleat it neatly in an agitated sort of way.

Another resident whose needs were unattended was Fred. He had a very bad chest infection and sat for much of the afternoon on his own with just the occasional and very brief interaction with staff.

Quality Improvement

Those present came up with some very positive ways of improving practice. Firstly there was Alice. She enjoys being with her friend, Gerty, who plays dominoes quite well. The suggestion was that she could be included in the social interaction that was taking place during the game without the pressure to 'think' and select the correct tile.

It was also noted in relation to this episode that the casual nurse did not have any understanding of dementia. Staff said that this was common with other agency nursing staff. For the present it was seen to be the responsibility of senior staff to briefly explain the limitations of someone who is living with dementia. Another request was that the behaviour codes and descriptions of Personal Detractions be placed in the office of the unit.

One of the greatest improvements emerged as a result of mindfulness of Personal Detractions. Residents were no longer left unattended while staff did their work. For example, one day when staff had less time to be with residents, one put on an old time music tape. Each of the AINs chatted with the residents, did a little jig with them or briefly sang with them as they passed through the room. There was certainly no need for a formal type program. These residents were involved in such a way that they would have scored A+3 or +5 for at least one hour.

Another result was that staff became much more aware of their own behaviour. If some forgot the impact of loud talking and laughing on the residents, one of them would remind the other that they were being 'a bit noisy'!

Dementia Care Mapping certainly raised the awareness of the staff. Moments of 'free' time that a staff member had were used to support the residents. Increasingly residents had company whenever there was a need. And so, one resident helped push the crockery trolley over to the main kitchen. Another went with an AIN to collect the laundry trolley. On another occasion Vera, who was very distressed and calling out loudly, was taken for a walk in the garden in a wheelchair. Those just sitting in the dining room were soon joined by an AIN whether to converse, play games or browse through the newspaper or magazine. As well as the programs they themselves ran, AINs became more frequent assistants during my time with the residents. It was great to have the support, and to see the residents become more involved through spontaneous comments, laughter and active participation in exercises, games, discussions and music and all those other undemanding activities that help people with dementia experience a meaningful existence.

Date: 15/08/2002 Time 14:30–16.30 period: 2 Hours # Participants 8 # Staff: 2.5 # Residents 10 Observers: Marolyn Seaman & Sister Margaret Randall

Participant's Name	Time	14:35	14:40	14:45	14:50	14:55	15:00	15:05	15:10	15:15	15:20	15:25	15:30	15:35	15:40	15:45	15:50	15:55	16:00	16:05	16:10	16:15	16:20	16:25	16:30	ΣWIB / ΣTF
Lilly	BCC	K	K	K	A	F	K	N	N	N	W	A	K	N	/	B	N	X	X	N	X	/	/	N	K	+12
	WIB	+1	+1	+1	+1	+1	+1	+1	+1	+1	+1	-1	-1	+1	/	+1	+1	/	/	+1	/	/	/	+1	-1	18
Gerty	BCC	X	X	X	X	X	P	A	O	F	F	F	A	A	G	A	E	G	G	A	G	/	/	G	G	+33
	WIB	/	/	/	/	/	+1	+1	+1	+1	+1	+1	+1	+1	+3	+3	+1	+3	+3	+3	+3	/	/	+3	+3	17
Vera	BCC	M	M	B	M	B	M	M	F	F	F	F	F	F	F	F	F	F	F	F	F	/	/	F	F	+24
	WIB	+1	+1	+1	+1	+1	+1	+1	+1	+1	+1	+1	+1	+1	+1	+1	+3	+1	+1	+1	+1	/	/	+1	+1	22
Alice	BCC	/	/	/	/	/	F	E	E	E	S	E	A	A	G	G	A	G	/	/	/	/	/	G	G	+10
	WIB	/	/	/	/	/	+1	+3	+3	+3	+1	+3	+3	+1	-1	-1	-1	-1	/	/	/	/	/	-1	-3	14
Fred	BCC	/	/	/	/	/	U	F	F	U	U	U	U	U	U	U	K	U	U	U	U	/	/	U	V	-23
	WIB	/	/	/	/	/	-1	+1	+1	-1	-1	-1	-1	-1	-1	-1	-3	-3	-3	-3	-3	/	/	-3		15
Pam	BCC	/	C	A	Y	T	B	B	B	F	F	F	M	M	B	M	M	A	B	B	A	A	A	A	A	+29
	WIB	/	-1	+1	+1	+1	+1	+1	+1	+1	+1	+1	+1	+1	+1	+1	+1	+1	+1	+1	+1	+3	+3	+3	+1	23
Mollie	BCC	K	U	T	U	T	U	A	A	U	U	F	K	U	U	K	U	U	U	A	V	V	V	A	G	+3
	WIB	-1	-1	+1	-1	+3	-1	+1	+3	-1	-1	+1	-1	-1	-1	-1	-1	-1	-3	+3	/	/	+3	+3		21
Jack	BCC	K	A	K	K	T	B	A	B	F	F	B	B	B	A	P	P	P	P	G	G	G	G	G	G	+42
	WIB	+1	+1	+1	+1	+3	+1	+1	+1	+1	+1	+1	+1	+1	+1	+3	+3	+1	+1	+3	+3	+3	+3	+3	+3	24

WHERE PERSON-CENTRED CARE'S A GIVEN

ENGLAND

PENNY GARNER from Burford, Oxfordshire, describes how DCM has been developed into the SPOT (SPECAL Observational Tracking) system

All members of the current SPECAL team trained in DCM at Bradford, and an individualised form of DCM known as SPOT, (SPECAL Observational Tracking) has been under development at Burford since 1993. SPOT is thoroughly grounded in person-centred dementia care and DCM, and is now at the point of being formally written up.

This map took place in the SPECAL Unit at the former Burford Community Hospital on a Friday. The Friday Group is the name of the original EMI day service offered by the NHS when SPECAL first began work at Burford in 1990. All NHS services were withdrawn in May 2000, but the SPECAL team has been allowed to remain in occupation, and the Friday Group is now the flagship service within the SPECAL model of care development at Burford.

Person-centred care is a given within the Burford model, and all SPECAL care is first developed on an individual basis before being tested out in a communal setting. There may be many 'rooms within a room' operating at the Friday Group at any one time, and the raw data (narrative only) sheets can be processed in a variety of ways, including:

• producing a conventional DCM map to show the high WIB values and low incidence of Personal Detractions which can be sustained when person-centred care is a given.

• evaluating the WIB value profile of the Friday Group as an entity, as if it were itself a SPECAL client

• developing and refining personalised BCCs (known as SPOT Indices – SPOTIs) for individual clients

• developing risk management strategies which address both emotional and physical risk factors

• developing Continuity of Acceptable Recycled Experience (CARE) on a 24 hour basis which may then itself be recycled on a lifelong basis.

The SPECAL approach aims to promote a lifelong continuity of acceptable experience. It makes the assumption that since comparatively few new experiences are remembered by people with dementia, while certain pre-dementia experiences are remembered in certain circumstances, pleasurable routines may be recycled without risk of boredom to the person with dementia. Further, it is assumed that if a person does not readily obtain individually relevant and personally acceptable information (either from self or others) when this is needed, then personhood and a sense of well-being will not be sustained. It is therefore considered crucial to know how to assess acceptability moment by moment as information is relayed, and to know when it is safe to avoid disturbing the sense that is

being made of any particular moment. SPOT is therefore needed by the carer of the moment, as part of the development of continuity of acceptable recycled experience (CARE).

Key developments of SPOT

1. Raw data sheet comprises continuous narrative notes on a second by second basis, to inform later completion of grid at a more leisurely pace.

2. BCCs have been broadly divided as follows:

(AH) to indicate active holding by a second person

(PH) to indicate passive holding by an activity without the involvement of others

(P/AQ) to indicate questioning of self or others, spoken or unspoken

2. BCCs include one additional category Q - Questioning of either self or others

3. WIB scoring has been simplified to reflect values which are either acceptable or unacceptable to the person, whilst including an additional factor to indicate whether WIB is rising or falling or static within the time frame

4. Time frames have been expanded to cover periods of 60 seconds or less

5. Processing of raw data sheet provides various indicators of progress towards the development of 24 hour CARE which may then itself be recycled on a lifelong basis.

6. Findings may be further analysed within the wider context of a conventional DCM exercise and used to inform Risk Management Strategies.

7. Personal Detractions have been extended to include a new category of 'Laying Mines' – drawing unnecessarily on the recent, and therefore problematic, experience of the person. Laying Mines is the PD most frequently recorded by SPOT.

What you see in the map

The map covers a period of approximately two hours and includes evidence of:

• A portrait in words of the activities of the Friday Group on one particular day

• The staggered introduction of clients into the room

• The changing of props in the room to make way for restaurant style lunch without disruption

• The use of ancillary staff to interact meaningfully with clients

• The investment of intensive one-to-one engagement leading to passively sustained activities

• Rooms within a room which can merge and move apart

• The use of furniture position as a care development prop.

My best experience with DCM was mapping a lady who burst into tears, apparently without reason, every day at about 12.0 noon in the Day Centre. Mapping revealed that she perceived any staff moving about the room as potentially 'visiting' her, and she was meeting with unattended distress on each occasion as they failed to pick up on her anticipatory body language. Each time her WIB value rose only to fall, and after this had happened about four times she was well on her way to drowning in a sea of disappointment, which finally manifested itself as tears by about noon. One mapping session of three hours was all that was needed to rectify the situation in a most dramatic way the next week.

My worst experience with DCM was being called in by the mental health services to map a resident in a local nursing home, who was being extraordinarily disruptive in that setting yet calm and focussed on creative activities within the Friday Group. I set up the session up in advance, with full support from the CPN, only to be refused entry on the day by the nursing home staff. The resident was withdrawn from the Friday Group and died shortly afterwards.

Date: 13.9.02 Time Period: 10.15 – 12.30 Place: Burford No. Participants: No. Staff: Observer: Penny Garner

Participant Name	Time	10.15	10.20	10.25	10.30	10.35	10.40	10.45	10.50	10.55	11.00	11.05	11.10	11.15	11.20	11.25	11.30	11.35	11.40	11.45	11.50	11.55	12.00	12.05	12.10	12.15	12.20	12.25	12.30		ΣWIB / ΣTF
RB	BCC	A	I	I	I	I	I	I	F	I	I	L	L	I	L	L	L	L	L	L	L	L	K	A	A	F	A	A			
	WIB	+3	+3	+3	+3	+3	+3	+3	+3	+3	+3	+3	+3	+3	+3	+3	+3	+3	+3	+3	+3	+3	+3	+5	+5	+3	+3	+3			
TT	BCC	A	I	A	A	A	A	A	F	L	L	L	L	L	L	L	L	L	L	L	A	L	L	L	K	K	B	A	F		
	WIB	+3	+3	+5	+5	+3	+5	+5	+1	+3	+3	+3	+3	+5	+3	+5	+3	+3	+3	+3	+3	+3	+3	+5	+5	+1	+5	+3	+3		
RD	BCC									O	F	O	F	F	L	I	L	L	L	A	A	A	A	B	B	B	B	F	F		
	WIB									+3	+1	+1	+1	+1	+1	+1	+1	+5	+5	+1	+3	+1	+1	+5	+1	+1	+1	+1	+1		
VS	BCC											E	E	E	E	E	E	E	A	H	H	H	A	A	A	A	F	F	F		
	WIB											+5	+3	+5	+5	+5	+5	+5	+5	+3	+3	+3	+5	+1	+1	+5	+3	+3	+3		
CM	BCC												A	A	A	A	E	E	A	E	E	A^Q	A^Q	A^Q	A^Q	A^Q	F	F	F		
	WIB												+5	+5	+5	+5	+5	+5	+5	+5	+5	+5	+5	+5	+5	+5	+3	+3	+3		
BS	BCC																K	A	A	A	A	A	A	A	A	F	F	F	F		
	WIB																+5	+5	+5	+5	+5	+5	+5	+1	+1	+3	+3	+3	+3		
JF	BCC																		K	A	A	A	A	A	A	F	F	F	F		
	WIB																		+5	+5	+5	+5	+5	+1	+1	+3	+3	+3	+3		

GIVING IT IN BLACK AND WHITE

FINLAND

SALIA SORMUNEN & PAÏVI TOPO explain how they have used mapping in Finland. They indicate how feedback was given following a mapping observation

We have been mapping since August 2001. This map took place in a hospital ward giving dementia care.

We considered the results with a dementia expert and looked at the recommendations, both for each individual and for the whole unit. We then gave verbal and written feedback to staff. In follow-up mapping we used the results of the first mapping as a basis to show how the situation had changed.

We knew the diagnosis, MMSE score and something of the daily habits of all the people we mapped. We were able to read the notes for each individual in the unit.

In our first mapping in the ward we saw that even if there were some activities residents spend quite a lot of time sitting quietly. This was the case especially among most passive/silent residents. On the other hand there was quite a lot of interaction between the residents. The third main issue we saw was that if some organised activity was going on there needed to be at least one staff member involved all the time, otherwise the well-being of the participants decreased quickly. In general, mapping showed quite positive results and the variance between the well-being of the individuals.

Our best experience with DCM was our first feedback session to staff in the observed unit. The DCM results prompted good discussion between staff members about the people who had been observed. A dementia expert was also present in the session; she offered her knowledge on dementia and care of people with dementia. Her role was quite important in stimulating the discussion about the results and in showing ways to improve care. Staff seemed very pleased to have the opportunity to discuss their clients with an experienced outsider and the mappings we had done provided a good basis for the discussion. This was also reported in the feedback questionnaire for the staff.

Some nurses became very nervous when being mapped. To map in that kind of situation is uncomfortable for both sides. It is not easy to describe Personal Detractions when you remember quite well which nurse was involved in the situation and that person is present in the feedback session.

The most difficult mapping was to map a person who has very difficult behavioural problems: she was walking nearly non-stop and lay down on the floor to rest some minutes; she was not able to talk any more but was crying and whimpering. She got very individual care but it was difficult to map her well-being. Her diagnosis was Lewy body disease.

The Personal Detractions that we have observed most often are invalidation and ignoring.

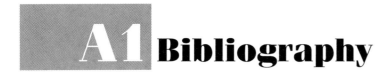 **Bibliography**

Research Papers, Descriptive/Discussion papers, Books and Reports

Adams, T. (1996). Kitwood's approach to dementia and dementia care: a critical but appreciative review. *Journal of Advanced Nursing*, 23: 948-953.

Agger, C. and Bonde Nielsen, E. (2001) *Kvalitetssikring af omsorg for svage aeldre: Pilotafprovning af DCM-metoden, Dementia Care Mapping, i Danmark*. Kobenhavns Kommune Sundhedsforvaltningen, Danie – Danmarks Institut for Aeldrepaedagogik. Copenhagen.

Audit Commission (2000). *Forget Me Not. Mental Health Services for Older People*. London. Audit Commission.

Baker, C. (2002). Is it really such a risk? *Journal of Dementia Care*, 10(2) 8.

Ballard, C., Fossey, J., Chithramohan, R., Howard, R., Burns, A., Thompson, P., Tadros, G. and Fairbairn, A. (2001) Quality of care in private sector and NHS facilities for people with dementia: cross sectional survey. *British Medical Journal*, 323: 426-427.

Ballard C., O'Brien J., James, I., Mynt, P., Lana, M., Potkins, D., Reichelt, K., Lee, L., Swann, A., and Fossey, J. (2001) Quality of life for people with dementia living in residential and nursing home care: the impact of performance on activities of daily living, behavioral and psychological symptoms, language skills and psychotropic drugs. *International Psychogeriatrics*, 13: 93-106.

Ballard, C., O'Brien, J., Swann, A., Fossey, J. and Lana, M. A One Year Follow-up study of behavioural and psychological symptoms in dementia (BPSD) amongst people in care environments. *Journal of Clinical Psychiatry* (In Press).

Barnett, E. (2000) *Including the Person with Dementia in Designing and Delivering Care - 'I need to be me!'*. Jessica Kingsley Publishers. London and Philadelphia.

Barnett, E. (1995) A window of insight into quality of care. *Journal of Dementia Care*, 3(4) 23-26.

Beavis, D. (1998) Personal detractions – a personal account. *Journal of Dementia Care*. 6(4) 24-25.

Beavis, D., Simpson, S, and Graham, I. (2002) A literature review of dementia care mapping: methodological considerations and efficacy. *Journal of Psychiatric and Mental Health Nursing*.9: 725-36.

Bolton, J., Gee, I., Jackson, L., Mather, D., Potter, L., Roberts, S., Robson, P., Scurfield, M., Stewart, D. and Vandor, C. (2000) Stepping back to move forward with DCM. *Journal of Dementia Care*, 4(4) 26-28.

Bredin, K., Kitwood, T. and Wattis, J. (1995) Decline in quality of life for patients with severe dementia following a ward merger. *International Journal of Geriatric Psychiatry*, 10: 967-973.

Brooker, D. (2003) Maintaining Quality in Dementia Care Practice, pp 240-255. In T. Adams and J. Manthorpe (Eds), *Dementia Care*, Arnold, London.

Brooker, D. (2002) Dementia Care Mapping: a look at its past, present and future. *Journal of Dementia Care*. 10(3) 33-36.

Brooker, D. (2001) Enriching Lives: evaluation of the ExtraCareActivity Challenge. *Journal of Dementia Care*, 9(3) 33-37.

Brooker, D. (2000) The Quality of Formal Care Services for People with Dementia. In G. Corley (Ed.) *Elderly People and their Needs*. Whurr Publications.

Brooker, D. (1999) DCM and Engagement combined to audit care quality. *Journal of Dementia Care*, 7(3) 33-36.

Brooker, D. (1995) Looking at them, looking at me. *Journal of Mental Health*, 4: 145-156.

Brooker, D. and Duce, L. (2000) Wellbeing and activity in dementia: a comparison of group reminiscence therapy, structured goal-directed group activity and unstructured time. *Aging & Mental Health*, 4 (4): 354-358.

Brooker D., and Payne M. (1995) Auditing outcome of care in in-patient and day patient settings using dementia care mapping. Can it be done? *PSIGE Newsletter,* No. 51 December 1994 - January 1995: 18-22.

Brooker, D., Foster, N., Banner, A., Payne, M. and Jackson, L. (1998) The efficacy of Dementia Care Mapping as an audit tool: report of a 3-year British NHS evaluation. *Aging & Mental Health*, 2 (1): 60-70.

Bruce, E., Surr, C. and Tibbs, M.A. (2002) *A Special Kind of Care. Improving Well-being in People Living With Dementia*. MHA Care Group. Derby. Available on the web at www.mha.org.uk

Cox, S. (2001) Developing quality in services. In C. Cantley (ed.) *A Handbook of Dementia Care*. Open University Press, Buckinghamshire.

Ford, J., King, M., Powell, J., Herzberg, J. (2003) Clinical Audit – a powerful tool to optimise care. *Journal of Dementia Care*. 11(6) 20-21.

Fossey, J.(1999) A carer on the team. *Journal of Dementia Care*, 7(2) 10.

Fossey, J., Lee, L., Ballard, C. (2002) Dementia Care Mapping as a research tool for measuring quality of life in care settings: psychometric properties. *International Journal of Geriatric Psychiatry*, 17: 1064 – 1070.

Fox, L. (1995) Dementia Care Mapping. *Care Home Management Bulletin*, Issue 9.

Fox, L. (1995) Mapping the advance of the new culture in dementia care pp 70-74. In *The New Culture of Dementia Care*. T. Kitwood and S.Benson (eds). Hawker Publications, London.

Harr, R. and Kasayka, R. (2000) The power of place and the preservation of personhood. *Nursing Homes: Long Term Management*, June, Vol 9. No. 6: 30-35.

Innes, A. (Ed), (2003) *Dementia Care Mapping: Applications Across Cultures*. Health Professions Press. Maryland.

Innes, A. (2002) Dementia Care Mapping: A useful method for Social Work? *Practice* 14 (1): 27-38

Innes, A. (2000) Dementia Care Mapping pp 112-122. In *Innovativer Umgang mit Dementen: Strategien, Konzepte und Einrichtungen in Europa*. H. SträBer and M. Cofone (Eds), Saarlouis

Innes, A., Capstick, A. and Surr, C. (2000) Mapping out the framework. *Journal of Dementia Care*, 8(2) 20-21.

Innes, A., Capstick, A. and Surr, C. (1999) Warning on DCM and Engagement methods, Letter to editor. *Journal of Dementia Care*, 7(4) 20-21.

Innes, A. and Surr, C. (2001) Measuring the well-being of people with dementia living in formal care settings: the use of Dementia Care Mapping. *Aging & Mental Health*, 5(3): 258-268.

Jacques, I. (1996) Evaluating care services for people living with dementia. *Elderly Care* June/July. Vol 8, No. 3.

James, I., Lee, L., Sells, K. and Allen, B. (2002) Quality of Care: Are we painting too black a picture? *Journal of Dementia Care*, 10(1) 37-38.

Kitwood, T. (1997) *Dementia Reconsidered: the Person Comes First*. Open University Press, Buckingham: .

Kitwood, T. (1993) Person and process in dementia. *International Journal of Geriatric Psychiatry*, 8: 541-545.

Kitwood, T. (1992) Quality assurance in dementia care. *Geriatric Medicine*, 22: 34-38.

Kitwood, T. and Benson, S. (Eds.), (1995) *The New Culture of Dementia Care*. Hawker Publications, London.

Kitwood, T. and Bredin, K. (1994) Charting the course of quality care. *Journal of Dementia Care*, 2(3) 22-23.

Kitwood, T. and Bredin, K. (1992) A new approach to the evaluation of dementia care. *Journal of Advances in Health and Nursing Care*, 1:5: 41-60.

Kitwood, T., Buckland, S. and Petre, T. (1995) *Brighter Futures: A report on research into provision for persons with dementia in residential homes, nursing homes and sheltered housing*. Anchor Housing Association.

Kuhn, D. and Verity, J. (2002) Putdowns and uplifts: signs of good or poor dementia care. *Journal of Dementia Care* 10(5) 26-27.

Kuhn D., Kasayka R, and Lechner C. (2002). Behavioral observations and quality of life among residents with dementia in ten assisted living facilities. *The American Journal of Alzheimer's Disease* 17(5) 291-298.

Kuhn, D., Ortigara, A. and Kasayka, R. (2000) Dementia Care Mapping: An innovative tool to measure person-centered care. *Alzheimer's Care Quarterly*, 1(3) 7-15.

Lechner, C. (2001) Dementia Care Mapping: A new approach to Alzheimer's Care. *Rehab & Community Care Management*, Fall: 40-42.

Lintern, T., Woods, R. and Phair, L. (2000a) Before and after training: a case study of intervention. *Journal of Dementia Care*, 8(1) 15-17.

Lintern, T., Woods, R. and Phair, L. (2000b) Training is not enough to change care practice. *Journal of Dementia Care*, 8(2) 15-17.

Mackenzie, L., James, I.A. and Lee, L. (2002) How DCM feedback procedures can be improved. *Journal of Dementia Care* 10(5) 23-25.

Maguire, S. and Gosling, A-L. (2003) Social and sensory stimulation groups: do the benefits last? *Journal of Dementia Care* 11(2) 20-22.

Martin, G.W. and Younger, D. (2001) Person-centred care for people with dementia: a quality audit approach. *Journal of Psychiatric and Mental Health Nursing* 8(5) 443-448.

Martin, G. and Younger, D. (2000) Anti oppressive practice: a route to the empowerment of people with dementia through communication and choice. *Journal of Psychiatric and Mental Health Nursing*, 7: 59-67.

Moyes, M., and Christie, H. (1998) Focus on each individual's experience and emotions. *Journal of Dementia Care* 6(4) 16 - 18

Moyes M, Christie H (1998b) Structuring groups to make psychotherapy possible. *Journal of Dementia Care* 6(5) 15-17.

Neel, A. (2002) How DCM may affect caregiver mappers. *Journal of Dementia Care*, 10(4) 26-28.

Niebergall, C. (2002) Validation nach Feil und das Dementia Care Mapping. Zwei Methoden zur Verbesserung der Liebensqualität von Menschen mit einer Demenzerkrankung in der Psychogeriatrie des Tertianum Neutal in Berlingen TG. *Medical Journal*. Dezember 2002.

Packer, T. (2000) Series - Obstacles to Person-Centred Care Delivery. Part 3: Pass the hot potato - is this person-centred teamwork? *Journal of Dementia Care*, 8(5) 17-19.

Packer, T. (2000) Series - Obstacles to Person-Centred Care Delivery Part 2: Facing up to the Bills. *Journal of Dementia Care*, 8(4) 30-33.

Packer, T. (2000) Series - Obstacles to Person-Centred Care Delivery Part 1: Does Person-Centred Care exist? *Journal of Dementia Care*, 8(3) 19-21.

Packer, T. (1999) Worldwide spread of the new culture of care. *Journal of Dementia Care*,7(1) 14-16.

Packer, T. (1996) Shining a light on simple, crucial details. Journal of Dementia Care, 4(6) 22-23.

Packer, T. and Jeffries, M. (1997) Haloperidol, Hips and Toenails...(Person Centred Care Series). *Journal of Dementia Care*, 5(6) 22-24.

Perrin, T. (1999) Time to take a fresh look at Dementia Care Mapping. Letter to the Editor. *Journal of Dementia Care*, 7(5) 8.

Perrin T. (1998) Lifted into a world of rhythm and melody. *Journal of Dementia Care* 6(1) 22-24.

Perrin T. (1997) Occupational need in severe dementia. *Journal of Advanced Nursing* 25 934-941.

Perrin T. (1997) The Positive Response Schedule for Severe Dementia. *Aging and Mental Health*, 1 (2): 184-191.

Perrin, T. and May, H. (2000) *Wellbeing in Dementia: An Occupational Approach for Therapists and Carers*. Churchill Livingstone. London.

Persaud, M.and Jaycock, S. (2001) Evaluating Care Delivery: The application of dementia care mapping in learning disability residential services. *Journal of Learning Disabilities*, 5 (4): 345-352.

Pritchard, E. J. and Dewing, J. (2001) A multi-method evaluation of an independent dementia care service and its approach. *Aging and Mental Health*, 5 (1): 63-72.

Sabat, S. (1994) Excess disability and malignant social psychology: A case study of Alzheimer's Disease. *Journal of Community & Applied Social Psychology*, Vol 4: 157-166.

Sormunen, S., Topo, P., Eloniemi-Sulkava, U. and Voutilainen, P. (2002) Can Dementia Care Mapping provide a new means for evaluation of care given to people with dementia? *Gerontologia*, 16(3): 120-130.

Surr, C. and Bonde Nielsen, E. (2003) Inter-rater reliability in Dementia Care Mapping. *Journal of Dementia Care* 11(6) 33-35.

Surr, C. and Brooker, D. (2002) The Effects of Undertaking a DCM Training Course on Care Practice. *Signpost*. 7 (2): 16-18.

Vila-Miravent, J. (2001) *L'atenció integral a persones amb demència en centres residencials*. Collegi Oficial de Psicòlegs de Catalunya, 20(142): 8-10.

Wilkinson A.M. (1993) Dementia Care Mapping: A pilot study of its implementation in a psychogeriatric service. *International Journal of Geriatric Psychiatry*, 8: 1027-1029.

Williams J. and Rees J. (1997) The use of 'dementia care mapping' as a method of evaluating care received by patients with dementia: an initiative to improve quality of life. *Journal of Advanced Nursing*, 25: 316-323.

Wylie, K., Madjar, I. and Walton, J. (2002) Dementia Care Mapping: A person-centred approach to improving the quality of care in residential settings. *Geriaction*, 20 (2), 5-9.

Younger, D., Martin, G.W. (2000) Dementia Care Mapping: an approach to quality audit of services for people with dementia in two health districts. *Journal of Advanced Nursing*, 32(5), 1206 1212.

Bradford Dementia Group Publications

Bradford Dementia Group (1997) *Evaluating dementia care: The DCM Method*, 7th Edition, University of Bradford. (available only as part of basic DCM course)

Brooker, D. and Rogers, L. (Eds.) (2001) DCM *Think Tank Transcripts* 2001. University of Bradford.

Theses

Barnett, E. (1996). *I need to be me! A thematic evaluation of a dementia care facility based on the client perspective*. Doctoral Thesis, University of Bath, United Kingdom.

Brooker, D. (1998). *Improving the quality of care for people with dementia*. Doctoral Thesis, University of Birmingham, United Kingdom.

Greatorex, B. (2002) *The Structure of Well-being in Dementia*. Doctoral Thesis in Clinical Psychology, University of Leicester, United Kingdom.

Lintern, T.C. (2001) *Quality in Dementia Care: Evaluating Staff Attitudes and Behaviour*. Doctoral Thesis, University of Wales, Bangor, United Kingdom.

Lintern, T.C. (2002) *The perceptions of nursing home staff towards people with dementia and their care: A qualitiative exploration of care staff views prior to and following a period of training and development interventions*. Doctoral Thesis, Salomons Centre for Applied Social and Psychological Development, Canterbury Christ Church University College, United Kingdom.

Rüsing, Detlef (2003): *Die Reliabilität und Validität des Beobachtungsinstruments 'Dementia Care Mapping' – Eine Literaturanalyse*. Dorsten (Verlag Ingrid Zimmerman) ISBN: 3-928568-42-6; ca.80 pages, DIN A4 Copytyp; 14_ + available from www.pflegen-mit-wissen.de

Wylie, K. (2000). *Valuing Sensation and Sentience in Dementia Care*. Doctoral Thesis, University of Newcastle, Australia.

A2 DCM Strategic Leads

Australia

Virginia Moore
Brightwater Care Group
2 Water Road
Inglewood
Western Australia 6052
Tel: 08 9202 2800
Fax: 08 9202 2801
Email: Virginiam@brightwatergroup.com

Denmark

Eva Bonde Nielson
Director
Daniee
The Danish National Institute for Elderly Education
Degnemose Alle 83
DK-2700 Brønshøj
Denmark
Tel: +45 3860 6091
Email: ebn@daniae.dk

Germany

Christian Müller-Hergl
Arnold-Bocklin-Strasse 27 OR: Meinwerk-Institut
4141   Giersmauer 35
Dortmund   33098 Paderborn
Germany   Germany
Tel: 05251 290830
Website: www.dcm-deutschland.de

Japan

Yutaka Mizuno
Director
Department of Research
Obu Dementia Care Research and Training Centre
3-294 Hantsuki-cho
Obu
Aichi
474-0037
Japan
Tel: +81 562 44 5551
Fax: +81 562 44 5831
email RVB003@wamnet.wam.go.jp

Switzerland

Carsten Niebergall
Tertianum ZfP
CH-8267 Berlingen
Kronenhof
Switzerland
Tel: 0041 52 762 5757
Email: zfp@tertianun.ch

United Kingdom

Dawn Brooker
Bradford Dementia Group
School of Health Studies
University of Bradford
Unity Building
25 Trinity Road
Bradford BD5 0BB
Tel +44 (0) 1274 235726
Email: D.J.Brooker@Bradford.ac.uk

United States

Roseann Kasayka
The Corinne Dolan Alzheimer Centre
Heather Hill Hospital
12340 Bass Lake Road
Chardon
Ohio 44024
USA
Tel: 440 285 4040
Fax: 440 285 4378
Email: rkasayka@heatherhill.org

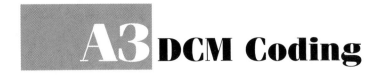

DCM Coding

Behaviour Category Coding

Code Memory	Cue	General description of category
A	Articulation	Interacting with others, verbally or otherwise (with no other obvious activity)
B	Borderline	Being socially involved, but passively
C	Cool	Being socially uninvolved, withdrawn
D	Distress	Unattended distress
E	Expression	Engaging in an expressive or creative activity
F	Food	Eating, drinking
G	Games	Participating in a game
H	Handicraft	Participating in a craft activity
I	Intellectual	Activity prioritising the use of intellectual abilities
J	Joints	Participating in exercise or physical sports
K	Kum and go	Independent walking, standing or wheelchair-moving
L	Labour	Performing work or work-like activity
M	Media	Engaging with media
N	Nod, land of	Sleeping, dozing
O	Own care	Independently engaging in self-care
P	Physical care	Receiving practical, physical or personal care
R	Religion	Participating in a religious activity
S	Sex	Activity related to explicit sexual expression
T	Timalation	Direct engagement of the senses
U	Unresponded to	Communicating without receiving a response
W	Withstanding	Repetitive self-stimulation
X	X-cretion	Episodes related to excretion
Y	Yourself	Talking to oneself, or an imaginary person
Z	Zero option	Behaviours that fit no existing category

Scale of well-being and ill-being

+5	exceptional well-being – it is hard to envisage anything better; very high levels of engagement, self-expression, social interaction
+3	considerable signs of well-being; for example in engagement, interaction or initiation of social contact
+1	coping adequately with present situation; some contact with others; no signs of ill-being observable
-1	slight ill-being visible; for example boredom, restlessness or frustration
-3	considerable ill-being; for example sadness, fear or sustained anger; moving deeper into apathy and withdrawal
-5	extremes of apathy, withdrawal, rage grief or despair

Personal Detraction Coding

Descriptions of forms of detractors

1. Treachery — using some form of deception in order to distract or manipulate a person, or force them into compliance.

2. Disempowerment — not allowing a person to use the abilities that they do have; failing to help them to complete actions that they have initiated.

3. Infantilization — treating a person very patronizingly (or 'matronizingly') as an insensitive parent might treat a very young child.

4. Intimidation — inducing fear in a person, through the use of threats or physical power.

5. Labelling — using a pattern of behaviour (e.g. smearer, stripper) or a category such as 'organic mental disorder', as the main basis for interacting with a person.

6. Stigmatization — treating a person as if they were a diseased object, an alien or an outcast.

7. Outpacing — providing information, presenting choices, etc, at a rate too fast for a person to understand; putting them under pressure to do things more rapidly than they can bear.

8. Invalidation — failing to acknowledge the subjective reality of a person's experience, and especially what they are feeling.

9. Banishment — sending the person away, or excluding them; physically or psychologically.

10. Objectification — treating a person as if they were a lump of dead matter, to be pushed, lifted, filled, pumped or drained, without proper reference to the fact that they are sentient beings.

11. Ignoring — carrying on (in conversation or action) in the presence of a person as if they were not there.

12. Imposition — forcing a person to do something, over-riding desire or denying the possibility of choice on their part.

13. Withholding — refusing to give asked for attention, or to meet an evident need; for example, for affectionate contact.

14. Accusation — blaming a person for actions or failures of action that arise from their lack of ability, or their misunderstanding of the situation.

15. Disruption — roughly intruding on a person's action or inaction; crudely breaking their 'frame of reference'.

16. Mockery — making fun of a person's 'strange' actions or remarks; teasing, humiliating, making jokes at their expense.

17. Disparagement — telling a person that they are incompetent, useless, worthless, etc; giving them messages that are damaging to their self esteem.

Scale: Mild (a)   Moderate (b)   Severe (c)   Very Severe (d)

Index